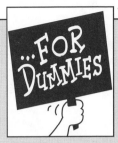

TM

# *References for the Rest of Us* ™

## BESTSELLING BOOK SERIES

Do you find that traditional reference books are overloaded with technical details and advice you'll never use? Do you postpone important life decisions because you just don't want to deal with them? Then our *...For Dummies®* business and general reference book series is for you.

*...For Dummies* business and general reference books are written for those frustrated and hard-working souls who know they aren't dumb, but find that the myriad of personal and business issues and the accompanying horror stories make them feel helpless. *...For Dummies* books use a lighthearted approach, a down-to-earth style, and even cartoons and humorous icons to dispel fears and build confidence. Lighthearted but not lightweight, these books are perfect survival guides to solve your everyday personal and business problems.

> **"More than a publishing phenomenon, 'Dummies' is a sign of the times."**
>
> **— The New York Times**

> **"...you won't go wrong buying them."**
>
> **— Walter Mossberg, Wall Street Journal, on IDG Books' ...For Dummies books**

> **"A world of detailed and authoritative information is packed into them..."**
>
> **— U.S. News and World Report**

**Already, millions of satisfied readers agree. They have made *...For Dummies* the #1 introductory level computer book series and a best-selling business book series. They have written asking for more. So, if you're looking for the best and easiest way to learn about business and other general reference topics, look to *...For Dummies* to give you a helping hand.**

D1531633

1/99

# The Weight Training Diary

## FOR DUMMIES®

## by Allen St. John

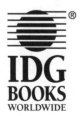

**IDG BOOKS WORLDWIDE**

IDG Books Worldwide, Inc.
An International Data Group Company

Foster City, CA ✦ Chicago, IL ✦ Indianapolis, IN ✦ New York, NY

**The Weight Training Diary For Dummies®**

Published by
**IDG Books Worldwide, Inc.**
An International Data Group Company
919 E. Hillsdale Blvd., Suite 300
Foster City, CA 94404
www.idgbooks.com (IDG Books Worldwide Web site)
www.dummies.com (Dummies Press Web site)

Library of Congress Control Number: 00-109312

ISBN: 0-7645-5336-4

Printed in the United States of America

10 9 8 7 6 5 4 3 2 1

1O/QV/QS/QR/IN

Distributed in the United States by IDG Books Worldwide, Inc.

Distributed by CDG Books Canada Inc. for Canada; by Transworld Publishers Limited in the United Kingdom; by IDG Norge Books for Norway; by IDG Sweden Books for Sweden; by IDG Books Australia Publishing Corporation Pty. Ltd. for Australia and New Zealand; by TransQuest Publishers Pte Ltd. for Singapore, Malaysia, Thailand, Indonesia, and Hong Kong; by Gotop Information Inc. for Taiwan; by ICG Muse, Inc. for Japan; by Intersoft for South Africa; by Eyrolles for France; by International Thomson Publishing for Germany, Austria and Switzerland; by Distribuidora Cuspide for Argentina; by LR International for Brazil; by Galileo Libros for Chile; by Ediciones ZETA S.C.R. Ltda. for Peru; by WS Computer Publishing Corporation, Inc., for the Philippines; by Contemporanea de Ediciones for Venezuela; by Express Computer Distributors for the Caribbean and West Indies; by Micronesia Media Distributor, Inc. for Micronesia; by Chips Computadoras S.A. de C.V. for Mexico; by Editorial Norma de Panama S.A. for Panama; by American Bookshops for Finland.

For general information on IDG Books Worldwide's books in the U.S., please call our Consumer Customer Service department at 800-762-2974. For reseller information, including discounts and premium sales, please call our Reseller Customer Service department at 800-434-3422.

For information on where to purchase IDG Books Worldwide's books outside the U.S., please contact our International Sales department at 317-572-3993 or fax 317-572-4002.

For consumer information on foreign language translations, please contact our Customer Service department at 1-800-434-3422, fax 317-572-4002, or e-mail rights@idgbooks.com.

For information on licensing foreign or domestic rights, please phone +1-650-653-7098.

For sales inquiries and special prices for bulk quantities, please contact our Order Services department at 800-434-4322 or write to the address above.

For information on using IDG Books Worldwide's books in the classroom or for ordering examination copies, please contact our Educational Sales department at 800-434-2086 or fax 317-572-4005.

For press review copies, author interviews, or other publicity information, please contact our Public Relations department at 650-653-7000 or fax 650-653-7500.

For authorization to photocopy items for corporate, personal, or educational use, please contact Copyright Clearance Center, 222 Rosewood Drive, Danvers, MA 01923, or fax 978-750-4470.

# About the Author

**Allen St. John** is the author of *Bicycling For Dummies* and *Skiing For Dummies* and is a former senior editor at *Condé Nast Women's Sports and Fitness* magazine. An avid recreational athlete, he has written about sports and fitness for a wide variety of national newspapers and magazines including *Men's Journal, MH-18, U.S. News & World Report, Maxim,* and the *New York Times.* He's a columnist for *Skiing* magazine, a regular contributor to *Tennis,* and a founding contributing editor for *Bike,* and he has covered the New York Yankees for the *Village Voice* for the past eight seasons as well as contributed to the hardcover book and CD-ROM, *The Way Baseball Works.* He lives in Upper Montclair, New Jersey, with his wife, Sally, and two children, Ethan and Emma.

# ABOUT IDG BOOKS WORLDWIDE

Welcome to the world of IDG Books Worldwide.

IDG Books Worldwide, Inc., is a subsidiary of International Data Group, the world's largest publisher of computer-related information and the leading global provider of information services on information technology. IDG was founded more than 30 years ago by Patrick J. McGovern and now employs more than 9,000 people worldwide. IDG publishes more than 290 computer publications in over 75 countries. More than 90 million people read one or more IDG publications each month.

Launched in 1990, IDG Books Worldwide is today the #1 publisher of best-selling computer books in the United States. We are proud to have received eight awards from the Computer Press Association in recognition of editorial excellence and three from Computer Currents' First Annual Readers' Choice Awards. Our best-selling ...For Dummies® series has more than 50 million copies in print with translations in 31 languages. IDG Books Worldwide, through a joint venture with IDG's Hi-Tech Beijing, became the first U.S. publisher to publish a computer book in the People's Republic of China. In record time, IDG Books Worldwide has become the first choice for millions of readers around the world who want to learn how to better manage their businesses.

Our mission is simple: Every one of our books is designed to bring extra value and skill-building instructions to the reader. Our books are written by experts who understand and care about our readers. The knowledge base of our editorial staff comes from years of experience in publishing, education, and journalism — experience we use to produce books to carry us into the new millennium. In short, we care about books, so we attract the best people. We devote special attention to details such as audience, interior design, use of icons, and illustrations. And because we use an efficient process of authoring, editing, and desktop publishing our books electronically, we can spend more time ensuring superior content and less time on the technicalities of making books.

You can count on our commitment to deliver high-quality books at competitive prices on topics you want to read about. At IDG Books Worldwide, we continue in the IDG tradition of delivering quality for more than 30 years. You'll find no better book on a subject than one from IDG Books Worldwide.

John Kilcullen
Chairman and CEO
IDG Books Worldwide, Inc.

*Eighth Annual Computer Press Awards ≥1992*

*Ninth Annual Computer Press Awards ≥1993*

*Tenth Annual Computer Press Awards ≥1994*

*Eleventh Annual Computer Press Awards ≥1995*

IDG is the world's leading IT media, research and exposition company. Founded in 1964, IDG had 1997 revenues of $2.05 billion and has more than 9,000 employees worldwide. IDG offers the widest range of media options that reach IT buyers in 75 countries representing 95% of worldwide IT spending. IDG's diverse product and services portfolio spans six key areas including print publishing, online publishing, expositions and conferences, market research, education and training, and global marketing services. More than 90 million people read one or more of IDG's 290 magazines and newspapers, including IDG's leading global brands — Computerworld, PC World, Network World, Macworld and the Channel World family of publications. IDG Books Worldwide is one of the fastest-growing computer book publishers in the world, with more than 700 titles in 36 languages. The "...For Dummies®" series alone has more than 50 million copies in print. IDG offers online users the largest network of technology-specific Web sites around the world through IDG.net (http://www.idg.net), which comprises more than 225 targeted Web sites in 55 countries worldwide. International Data Corporation (IDC) is the world's largest provider of information technology data, analysis and consulting, with research centers in over 41 countries and more than 400 research analysts worldwide. IDG World Expo is a leading producer of more than 168 globally branded conferences and expositions in 35 countries including E3 (Electronic Entertainment Expo), Macworld Expo, ComNet, Windows World Expo, ICE (Internet Commerce Expo), Agenda, DEMO, and Spotlight. IDG's training subsidiary, ExecuTrain, is the world's largest computer training company, with more than 230 locations worldwide and 785 training courses. IDG Marketing Services helps industry-leading IT companies build international brand recognition by developing global integrated marketing programs via IDG's print, online and exposition products worldwide. Further information about the company can be found at www.idg.com. 1/26/00

# Dedication

To my kids, Ethan and Emma, who do everything they can to keep me in shape.

# Author's Acknowledgments

Although there's one name on the cover, a book is a team effort. I'd like to thank everyone at IDG Books, including executive editor Stacy Collins and project editors Mike Kelly and Greg Summers, and of course my agent, the incomparable Mark Reiter, and the rest of the good people at IMG Literary. Special thanks go to this book's technical reviewer, Jeff Csatari, who helped make sure that the information in this book is as smart and accurate as it can be.

Thanks also to all the editors who help me make a living putting words together, including James Kaminsky, Albert Baime, and Alex Straus at *Maxim*, David Sparrow, James Martin, and Bill Gray at *Tennis*, Rick Kahl, Helen Olsson, Bevin Wallace, Mike Miracle, and Charlie Glass at *Skiing*, Dana White at *Teen People*, Brian Duffy at *U.S. News & World Report*, King Kaufman at *Salon.com*, Jerry Beilinson at *National Geographic Adventure*, Miles Seligman at the *Village Voice*, Michael Anderson at the *New York Times Book Review*, Jack Schwartz at the *New York Times*, Kyle Creighton at the *New York Times Magazine*, and, of course, anyone that I'm forgetting.

And finally to my wife, Sally, my support, my inspiration, and my best friend.

# Publisher's Acknowledgments

We're proud of this book; please register your comments through our IDG Books Worldwide Online Registration Form located at www.dummies.com.

Some of the people who helped bring this book to market include the following:

## Acquisitions, Editorial, and Media Development

**Project Editor:** Michael Kelly, Greg Summers

**Executive Editors:** Stacy S. Collins

**Copy Editor:** Robert Annis

**Acquisitions Coordinator:** Stacy Klein

**General Reviewer:** Jeff Csatari

**Editorial Manager:** Jennifer Ehrlich

**Editorial Administrator:** Michelle Hacker

**Cover Photos:**

Front Cover Carl Vanderschuit / FPG International

Back Cover Peter Magielsen / International Stock

## Production

**Project Coordinator:** Leslie Alvarez

**Layout and Graphics:** Amy Adrian, Joe Bucki, Jill Piscitelli, Jacque Schneider, Brian Torwelle, Julie Trippetti, Erin Zeltner

**Proofreaders:** Susan Moritz, Carl Pierce, York Production Services, Inc.

**Indexer:** York Production Services, Inc.

## General and Administrative

**IDG Books Worldwide, Inc.:** John Kilcullen, CEO; Bill Barry, President and COO; John Ball, Executive VP, Operations & Administration; John Harris, CFO

**IDG Books Consumer Reference Group**

**Business:** Kathleen A. Welton, Vice President and Publisher; Kevin Thornton, Acquisitions Manager

**Cooking/Gardening:** Jennifer Feldman, Associate Vice President and Publisher

**Education/Reference:** Diane Graves Steele, Vice President and Publisher; Greg Tubach, Publishing Director

**Lifestyles:** Kathleen Nebenhaus, Vice President and Publisher; Tracy Boggier, Managing Editor

**Pets:** Dominique De Vito, Associate Vice President and Publisher; Tracy Boggier, Managing Editor

**Travel:** Michael Spring, Vice President and Publisher; Suzanne Jannetta, Editorial Director; Brice Gosnell, Managing Editor

**IDG Books Consumer Editorial Services:** Kathleen Nebenhaus, Vice President and Publisher; Kristin A. Cocks, Editorial Director; Cindy Kitchel, Editorial Director

**IDG Books Consumer Production:** Debbie Stailey, Production Director

**IDG Books Packaging:** Marc J. Mikulich, Vice President, Brand Strategy and Research

◆

The publisher would like to give special thanks to Patrick J. McGovern, without whom this book would not have been possible.

◆

# Contents at a Glance

# Cartoons at a Glance

*By Rich Tennant*

The 5th Wave    By Rich Tennant

"Okay, I know I need to start working out. Now, can I please have my soap-on-a-rope back?"

*page 179*

The 5th Wave    By Rich Tennant

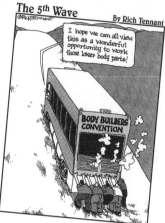

I hope we can all view this as a wonderful opportunity to work those lower body parts!

BODY BUILDERS CONVENTION

*page 7*

The 5th Wave    By Rich Tennant

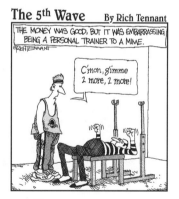

THE MONEY WAS GOOD, BUT IT WAS EMBARRASSING BEING A PERSONAL TRAINER TO A MIME.

C'mon, gimme 2 more, 2 more!

*page 55*

*Cartoon Information:*
*Fax:* 978-546-7747
*E-Mail:* richtennant@the5thwave.com
*World Wide Web:* www.the5thwave.com

# Table of Contents

# Introduction

● ● ● ● ● ● ● ● ● ● ● ● ● ● ● ● ● ● ● ● ● ● ● ● ● ● ● ● ● ● ● ● ● ● ● ● ● ● ● ● ● ● ● ● ●

*T*here's something very simple and almost magical about weight lifting. You pick up a weight; you put it down. Repeat as necessary. And tomorrow you find that today's sweat pays dividends. You discover that you can lift a heavier weight — or maybe lift the same one three more times. This book is about helping you toward those oh-wow moments when you find yourself able to do something that you never could before.

## About This Book

So you've decided to hide that bowl of nacho chips, pop the AAA batteries out of the remote, and get off the couch for good. Congratulations. But while that first step is important, the real key to getting in shape — and staying there — is consistency. Day after day, week after week, month after month, you need to make exercise as much a part of your day as brushing your teeth. And that's where this book comes in.

Part information source, part motivational tool, and part journal, this book will help you get started exercising, help you to get the most out of every workout, and, yes, even supply a gentle kick in the pants when your willpower flags. Not bad for a pile of paper that fits in your gym bag.

In these pages, you find out how to set up an exercise program that's just right for you. You discover how to warm up properly to prevent injuries. You get a wealth of workout tips in a variety of popular workout activities, from walking to swimming to in-line skating. Finally, you find out about how to cool down and recharge for your next workout.

And then comes the part of the book that you write yourself. The meat of this book is a customizable workout log where you can list your personal goals and record your progress. It's this section that makes this book truly *your* book.

And finally, because everyone loves a list, the Part of Tens, which gives you a few more tips and even a couple of jokes.

# Why You Should Log Your Workouts

First, here's what you shouldn't expect from this book. It won't improve your penmanship. It won't win you a Pulitzer Prize. And unless you win, say, a Nobel Prize or a presidential election on your own, it won't provide an insight into your personality for biographers of a future generation.

What logging your workouts does give you is pretty simple: motivation and information. First the motivation part. Have you ever made a to-do list? Have you ever made a to-do list after you've already completed the first three tasks, just so you get the satisfaction of crossing them off? Admit it, it's a great feeling. That's the same kind of reward that's waiting for you at the end of every exercise session.

The great thing about fitness is that it's quantifiable. Practice your new arrangement of "Afternoon Delight" on your Casiotone for a month, and you're depending on your friends to tell you how much better you sound. But when it comes to fitness, you're not dependent on the kindness of strangers. All you need to do is flip back through your training diary and realize that you're going farther and faster, or lifting more, than you did a month ago. Trust me, that's also a great feeling.

But unlike your old to-do lists, the completed pages of this training diary will also contain plenty of vital information. You'll see which goals were easy and fun to attain, and which goals made you feel like Wile E. Coyote chasing the Road Runner. By reviewing your entries, you'll be able to detect personal patterns and tendencies that will allow you to train more efficiently in the future. You'll also be able to improve your performance and prevent injuries. And, finally, you'll be able to have more fun . . . beyond the simple joy of seeing your accomplishments immortalized in black and white.

# How to Use Your Training Diary

The first thing you need to use your training diary is a pen. Got it? Good. The next thing you need is a plan. Before you start keeping a training diary, you should have a basic idea of what your fitness goals are and how to achieve them. (Don't worry, I talk about all that in Chapter 1.)

The next thing you need is a willingness to make your training diary your new friend. Bring this book with you to the gym, keeping it in your gym bag right next to your shower shoes. Or if you exercise outdoors, set it down on the kitchen counter, right next to a bottle of Gatorade, and make a beeline for it as soon as you get back from an exercise session. As soon as you've completed a workout, make it a habit to write down what you did and how you felt. If you record your workout right away, it's easy and fun. If you wait until later, it becomes a hassle. Or doesn't get done at all.

At the minimum, you should record how long you worked out, how many reps at each weight you did in the weight room, or the duration and distance of your aerobic workout. You might also record how you felt when you got up and before, during, and after your workout.

Because I know you're busy, this diary doesn't assume that you're going to work out every day of every week — in fact, a good workout plan includes a healthy balance of exercise and rest. With the diary section, you can track your progress over a ten-day stretch, customizing your journal each day for whatever workout you choose, running, weight training, and so on. And you can use the Training Goals section to write down your personal training goals and the Workout Wrap-Up section to celebrate your training accomplishments.

Finally, don't forget the Food for Thought section to track your diet and nutrition goals, as well as how you felt during your workout and what you should focus on for your next training session.

But this isn't a police report — your training diary can include anything that you feel is important. Did "99 Luftbaloons" keep running through your head on your bike ride? Did you finally figure out mid-rep why Ginger brought all those dresses for a three-hour tour? Did you step on the scale after your shower and finally see the needle settle at your target weight? Then write it down.

# Cheater, Cheater, Biscotti Eater

"When you cheat, you're only cheating yourself." Bet you haven't heard that one since grammar school. Well, I'm hear to tell you that Mrs. Moloney was right — about that, not about the fact that you'll never amount to anything unless you sit up straighter at your desk.

So while it's very tempting to write in on that first line — ran 7 miles / 42 minutes or bench press: 225 pounds — don't do it unless you really did it. First off, remember that this is a diary. And like the one with the poodle fur and the tiny gold key in which you promised your undying love to Jimmy Whatshisname, it's completely private. Your little sister won't read it unless you show it to her, so there's no need to hide it under the bed. Unless you decide to share it with your friends — or leave it for your biographer — no one's going to be impressed by what you wrote down, or think less of you if your workout was kind of lame.

So if you don't complete your planned workout on any given day, that's okay. Write down what you did and, if you can, why you think you fell short of your goal. Too tired? Too sore? Too little time? That info will help you down the road.

If you skip a couple of days of working out, that's okay, too. But if you start fudging and writing down miles not run and weights not lifted, you won't have an accurate yardstick of what you really did and how fast you really progressed. When you go back a couple of months later, you'll feel like a special prosecutor, trying to piece together who did what when. So take some sage advice from Samuel Langhorne Clemens — "When in doubt, tell the truth." Somewhere down the road, you'll be glad you did.

# How This Book Is Organized

Okay, this isn't *Anna Karenina* and I don't expect you to sit down with a bottle of vodka and a box of tissues and read it from start to finish. But this book does have a beginning, middle, and end. First off, you get a bit of sage advice. In the opening chapters, you find out how this book is organized — in fact that's what you're doing right now — how to plan a workout program, how to warm up properly, how to get the most out of your workout, and how to cool down and refuel for your next workout.

After that comes the place where you take center stage: the training diary pages. These pages give you a place to make a workout plan that's customized for your level of fitness, your goals, and your schedule. You also have a place to record each workout and monitor your progress. Each spread is complete with a fitness factoid or a quote guaranteed to pique your curiosity.

The book closes with the Part of Tens, a couple of short chapters filled with a few more amusing tips. And finally, the index will help you locate anything you can't find on your own.

# Icons Used in This Book

As with any *For Dummies* book, this one has icons to act as guideposts to special hints and notions along the way, each one offering a helpful perspective to consider as you plan your workout.

This icon highlights a quick hint that will help you train better and more efficiently.

Items flagged with this icon will help you to avoid accidents and injuries.

This icon is the graphic equivalent of a string tied around your finger, a reminder about something that you can't — or shouldn't — do without during your training or your race.

This icon flags training technique suggestions, workout gear recommendations, and fun facts you can use to amaze your friends at cocktail parties.

Information included with this icon offer suggestions that will make your workouts easier.

## Where to Go from Here

The important thing about training is to get started *today*. And start tracking your progress *today*. The sooner you start to make use of this book's diary and log your workout progress, the sooner you can see improvements in your daily training regimen. So turn the page (or use the Table of Contents or Index to get to the information you need the most) and get going!

# Part I
# The Training Basics

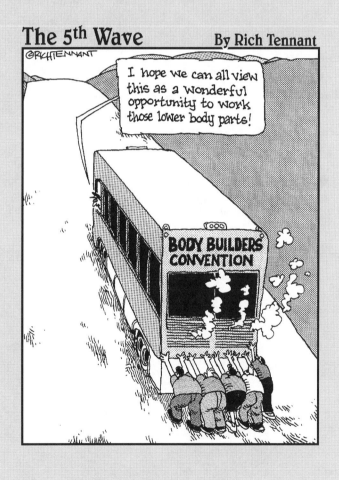

The 5th Wave                    By Rich Tennant

I hope we can all view this as a wonderful opportunity to work those lower body parts!

BODY BUILDERS CONVENTION

## In this part . . .

Ready to go? Good. But before you lace up your sneakers, pour yourself a cup of coffee, sit down, and spend a few minutes reading this section, where you'll learn how to get ready for a workout, train as efficiently as possible, and get ready for next time.

# Chapter 1

# Creating Your Workout Plan

● ● ● ● ● ● ● ● ● ● ● ● ● ● ● ● ● ● ● ● ● ● ● ● ● ● ● ● ● ● ● ● ● ● ● ● ● ● ● ● ● ● ●

*In This Chapter*

▶ Motivating yourself

▶ Finding time to work out

▶ Measuring your fitness

▶ Devising a workout plan

● ● ● ● ● ● ● ● ● ● ● ● ● ● ● ● ● ● ● ● ● ● ● ● ● ● ● ● ● ● ● ● ● ● ● ● ● ● ● ● ● ● ●

*W*hat do you have in common with a world class athlete and a James Bond supervillain? Each of you needs a plan. The good news is that you don't need to draw blood three times a day to check your lactate levels, and you don't need an evil laugh and a world map marking every missile silo to . . . *Ha Ha Hmmm . . . Rule the World!*

Even if you're not after a gold medal or global domination, but you simply want to lose a few pounds, a plan helps in any number of ways. It makes your workouts more efficient and helps you to see results more quickly.

Conversely, if you start a workout program without a plan, you're like that classic Sex Pistols song — don't know what you want, but you know how to get it.

## Why Exercise Anyway?

Before you delve into the whats, wheres, and hows of creating your own exercise program, back up and think about *why* you exercise in the first place. You probably know a lot of the answers, but listing them may just be the difference between getting up for that 6:30 workout or hitting the snooze button.

- **You'll be healthier:** By exercising, you can reduce your risk of serious and even life-threatening diseases such as diabetes, heart disease, and cancer. There's even evidence that exercise can ward off the common cold.

- **You'll look better:** Exercising not only burns calories but also boosts your metabolism, which makes it easier to maintain your desired weight without resorting to the celery and ice cream diet.

- **You'll be less stressed:** Exercise produces endorphins — the same mood-altering brain chemicals that are targeted by everything from chocolate to illicit drugs. Runner's high is more than a myth.

- **You'll have fun:** Remember when you used to go out and play after school, running and jumping, riding and skating until you were exhausted? Well, pick the right exercise and that same kind of fun is still there for the taking.

# Making Your Fitness Plan

If the road to fitness is a journey, then a fitness plan is your road map. You don't need to be a motivational guru to understand that before you can get in shape, you've got to identify some workout goals and figure out how to get from here to there.

First, you've got to identify your destination, or your goal. In this section, I tell you how to do that. Once you know where you're going, it becomes a lot easier to map out the shortest route there, which I discuss later in this chapter.

## Setting your fitness goals

In workouts and in life, goal setting can be both easy and hard. At its most basic level, setting a goal is as simple as identifying something you want. It can be as vague as, "I want to be happy." Or as specific as, "I want to be the executive vice president in charge of marketing by the end of September."

Workout-wise, you've got the same range of choices. Your objective can be as general as wanting to be healthier and feel better and have some fun. Or it can be as specific as saying, "I want to break 50 minutes in the Independence Day 10K." Or, "I want to drop 12 pounds and 2 dress sizes so that I'm looking good for Chris's wedding in August."

The bottom line is that the quality of the goal you set is directly proportional to your chance of achieving it. If your goal is too vague, it can be almost impossible to measure your progress. ("Do I really feel healthier and feel better than I did last week?")

If the goal is too specific, that can be a problem too. If you become too goal-oriented — "I've been exercising for three weeks and my time (or waistline) hasn't come down at all." — it's easy to get discouraged by slow progress or minor setbacks.

The best goals are those that have both macro and micro components. Your macro goal might be, "I want to run the New York City Marathon next year." Your micro goal might be, "I want to run the 5K in town faster than I did last year." In short, your everyday goal should be an easily achievable, bite-size chunk of that larger goal. The short-term goal gives you a reason to work out today — "The 5K is ten days away" is a much better incentive for getting out of bed than, say, "The marathon is ten months away."

## More than the standard disclaimer

My lawyers want me to tell you that you should consult your physician before beginning a program of physical exercise. Okay, there I said it. But I'd like this to sink in more than the seat-belt demonstration on an airliner. After all, you wouldn't take a car that's been in storage for five years straight to the drag strip, now would you?

Well, if your car deserves a trip to the mechanic, don't you deserve a trip to your friendly neighborhood physician. A pre-exercise physical exam can uncover some underlying problems — anything from heart disease to a blood sugar imbalance — that could be exacerbated by exercise. So do the right thing — go see your doctor.

And once you achieve that micro goal, you can pat yourself on the back, because you did what you set out to do, and you've also moved a little closer to your big objective. Which makes it easier to set another micro goal.

## Finding the time

The world's number-one all-purpose excuse? *I'm too busy.* Do you know anyone who's *not* too busy? I even hear it from my three-year-old son Ethan when I ask him to pick up his trains. "But, Daddy, I'm too busy." So let's find a way past the "B" word, shall we?

The first step is to make exercise a priority. Whether we write things down or not, every day each of us has a giant to-do list — with standing entries ranging from taking a shower to making enough money to pay the mortgage. So what you need to do is add one more thing that you absolutely, positively must do today: Get some exercise.

The best way to make sure that exercise becomes as automatic as brushing your teeth? Make it part of your schedule. Here are a few ways to incorporate exercise into your daily routine.

✔ **Do it early:** You remember Murphy's Law, right? Well, one of its axioms is that if you put off your workout until after work, and you go to the DMV, do grocery shopping, and drop the kids off at their friends' house, the following will happen. The DMV line will snake around the block, the baggers at the grocery store will stage a sitdown strike, and you'll get caught in a traffic jam on the way to the play date. In short, everything that can go wrong, will, and you'll be running an hour late, and today's workout will have to wait until tomorrow. If you work out first thing in the morning, you won't have to worry about life's little intrusions.

✔ **Multi-task:** Exercising can be tacked on to other chores, if you make it the first task, rather than the last. Stopping at the gym on your way to work, or right after you drop the kids off at school, is a great way to make sure that it gets done.

> ✔ **Get help:** Families and friends can place demands on you that can keep you from exercising. Or they can help clear your schedule so that you have the time. If you're having trouble finding time to exercise, talk to the people in your life. Whether it's trading chores to get a big enough block of time to go to the gym, or just asking for a little good-natured nagging — "So, lard butt, have you gone running yet or what?" — your significant others can lend a hand in helping you get into shape.

# Setting Up Your Workout Schedule

Now that you've identified some goals and carved out some time to exercise, the next step is to make a workout plan. Some of the benefits of having a workout plan are obvious.

If you've made a plan in advance, it eliminates what coaches call "game-time decision-making." It allows you to glance at the day's schedule and go out and do it, rather than trying to remember what your last workout was, and whether tomorrow's a rest day or not. Which means that you get out of the house and start breaking a sweat sooner.

But the biggest difference between having a workout plan and just going out and exercising is this: When you create a plan, you balance rest and recovery, and every workout has a specific purpose in helping you achieve your fitness goals. It's really about squeezing the maximum fitness benefit out of the minimum amount of time.

Build a smart plan and stick to it, and I guarantee you'll be stronger, fitter, and faster. And if after a month or two you can suddenly fit into a pair of jeans that you thought were two sizes too small, well, so much the better.

The first thing you need to do is determine how many days a week you're going to work out. If you're just starting out, three is a good number. And it's best to balance workout days with rest and recovery days (see Chapter 4 for more about the importance of rest). For that reason, you might start out by working out on Monday, Wednesday, and Friday. Or Tuesday, Thursday, and Saturday if that suits you better.

And if you're doing cross-training — combining two or more activities in your workout plan — then it makes sense to alternate your activities in addition to your workouts. For example, if you're going to ride your bike twice a week, swim once a week, and do one weight training session, your schedule might shake out like the one in Table 1-1.

### Table 1-1   A Typical Cross-Training Workout Schedule

| *Sun* | *Mon* | *Tue* | *Wed* | *Thu* | *Fri* | *Sat* |
|-------|-------|-------|-------|-------|-------|-------|
| Rest  | 30 min | Rest | 30 min |       | Rest  | 40 min | Rest  |
|       | Bike  |       | Swim + |       | Bike  |       |
|       |       |       | Resistance training |       |       |       |

The specifics aren't as important as the general principles. In Table 1-1, I alternate the rest and exercise days. The two bike rides are separated by two and three days, respectively, to give you ample time to recover. The duration of the workouts increases gradually through the week. And since you're going to the health club to swim, that's a good day to put in a few minutes in the weight room.

Of course, you can feel free to modify this plan to fit your schedule, your level of fitness, and your goals.

What about next week? In general, it's good to keep your schedule pretty much the same from week to week. Schedule the longer workouts and gym sessions on the same day, if possible. And while you should add to the length of the workouts, as your fitness level allows, don't push it too hard. Adding more than 10 percent a week is only inviting injury.

## *Getting into Training*

So you've already been doing this exercise thing for a while? Well, congratulations. Now may be the time for you to move from the land of the unstructured workout to full-fledged training.

Training? Don't get freaked out by the "T" word. Yeah, that's what athletes do, but in the end, your goals aren't really so much different from theirs. You want to get as fit as you can in as little time as possible, right? By focusing your training program, you can do just that.

## Measuring your fitness

Every good fitness program needs three good measuring tools. You've got one of the essentials right here in the form of this training diary. The other two you can buy at almost any sporting goods store — a watch with a stopwatch function and a heart-rate monitor. They form what a consultant might call a synergy.

- ✔ The watch tells you how long you worked out.

- ✔ The heart-rate monitor tells you how hard you worked.

- ✔ The training diary lets you keep track of your progress.

And all three together will motivate you to get out, identify your strengths and weaknesses, and help you get the most out of your training time.

While timing your workout is pretty basic, heart-rate monitoring was something that, until recently, only elite athletes did. At its most fundamental level, your heart rate is really the measuring stick of your cardiovascular fitness. If your speed goes up while your heart rate stays the same, then, congratulations, you're fitter. But even more importantly, your heart rate is the most reliable indicator of how your body is producing energy, which gives you the opportunity to target your training that much more accurately.

And while you can take your pulse by just putting a finger on an artery on your wrist or on your neck while you're exercising, it's far more convenient to just peek at your heart-rate monitor.

"But," you say, "I'm not an Olympic athlete." All the more reason why you need a heart-rate monitor. Olympic athletes actually have sort of a built-in heart-rate monitor, a sixth sense about how hard they're working, developed over years of training. They mostly use their heart-rate monitors to confirm what their bodies are already telling them.

## A buyer's guide to heart-rate monitors

A heart-rate monitor should have a readout that's big enough to read while you're exercising. The buttons should be big enough that you can manipulate them while you're on the go. The elastic chest strap, which actually takes the reading, should be comfortable both while you're at rest and while you're exercising. The most important function is the capability to set a target heart-rate range with an audible alarm that beeps when you're above or below it.

As for the more sophisticated programming options — anything from a post-workout readout of average heart rate to a full record of the workout that can be downloaded to your computer — let your love of gadgetry, or lack thereof, be your guide.

Ironically, recreational athletes, who can benefit most from a heart-rate monitor, are the least likely to own one. Newbies are more likely to judge their workout by speed rather than real workload, so they're likely to overdo it if they encounter a hill and loaf a little when they've got a tail wind.

Do you fall into that camp? Try this test: During your next workout, guess your heart rate. If you're not consistently within ten beats, you need a heart-rate monitor.

Having trouble getting a reading from your heart-rate monitor early in your workout? Try licking the sensor. Most rely on the conductivity of your sweat to work properly, and saliva is the best substitute.

## *Maxing out — speaking from the heart*

One bit of information that you need before you start a training program is your *maximum heart rate*. Throughout the rest of this chapter, different training intensities are expressed as a percentage of maximum heart rate. Here's the simplest way to determine your MHR:

> ✔ Women, subtract your age from 226. (A 33-year-old female would end up with a maximum heart rate of 193.)
>
> ✔ Men, subtract your age from 220. (A 33-year-old male calculates a maximum heart rate of 187.)

While this number should give you a reasonable ballpark rate, it doesn't take into account factors such as heredity and your present fitness level.

The other way of determining your maximum heart rate is by pushing yourself until you get there. The safest and most accurate way to do this is with a treadmill stress test administered by your doctor. And of course, before embarking on any exercise program, you should consult with your doctor.

# The Building Blocks of Training

So what's the difference between a planned workout and just plain exercising? Well, in a planned workout, you build at least one of three things: strength, speed, or endurance.

These are the building blocks of all fitness — whether it's on a bike, a basketball court, or a skating rink. Every sport more strenuous than chess calls upon these three basic qualities in various proportions. But before I talk about how to build your fitness, I need to define the terms.

## Endurance

Endurance is a pretty straightforward concept. It's the ability to run or ride or swim a little farther today than you did yesterday. Sure, some part of endurance is mental — it's a borderline obsessiveness that allows people to swim the English Channel or run an ultramarathon. But it's also physical attribute, the ability of your muscles and your connective tissues to keep going . . . and going . . . and going.

And for endurance efforts, your body produces energy *aerobically* — taking in as much oxygen as it's consuming — and uses fat as its primary fuel.

## Strength

Simply, strength is the ability to move mass, but it's more than just the ability to move a refrigerator or do 100 pushups. In most forms of exercise, whether it's swimming, running, or cycling, the mass that you're moving is, well, you. And improving your strength gives you the ability to move farther with every stride or stroke, as well as the ability to contend with natural obstacles such as head winds and hills.

For these kind of high-power activities, your body often functions *anaerobically* — you're consuming more oxygen than you can take in — and uses carbohydrates for quick energy.

## Speed

Speed is, you guessed it, the ability to move fast. And it's easy to measure, whether against a rival or against the clock. Simply, if you have any thoughts about competing, whether seriously or casually, you have the need for speed.

Speed workouts are usually highly anaerobic and use carbohydrate stores as a fuel source.

# The Three Kinds of Workouts

Okay, so you understand what your goals are. Now how do you tailor an aerobic program to increase your abilities? Well for starters, your master plan should incorporate three different kinds of workouts, each addressing one of the three cornerstones discussed in the preceding section.

## Long, steady distance

To improve your endurance, you're going to do *LSD* — long, steady distance — workouts. By building endurance, LSD workouts provide a base for your training schedule. They train your body to use fat as a fuel, which is the most efficient way to power your muscles for long-distance workouts. They also allow your body to recover from the stresses that your power- and speed-building workouts place on your body.

LSD workouts seem easy, and in a way, that's the problem. You feel like you should be doing more, and so you push yourself beyond the point at which you're getting maximum training benefit. Discipline yourself to go slowly and keep your heart rate in the target range. Shoot for between 50 and 70 percent of your maximum heart rate on LSD workouts.

## Strength training

While you can increase your strength by doing resistance workouts — running in sand, riding up hills, skating with really rusty bearings — the best way to get stronger is to hit the gym. A balanced whole-body program of weight lifting can increase your strength, help prevent injury, and even help you look better in a bathing suit.

It doesn't really matter whether you choose a machine-to-machine circuit or a series of light free-weight exercises. If you've never lifted weights before, ask a trainer at your gym or health club to show you proper form and help you design a workout plan. The key is stick-to-itiveness. It'll take about 12 to 16 weeks, working out two to three times a week, to really build your strength.

Unless your goal is to get pumped up Schwarzenegger-style, you should stay away from heavy weight/low rep exercises. Adding too much upper-body muscle could actually slow you down by adding a little power and a lot of extra weight.

## Speed intervals

To get fast, you need to do sprint intervals. The idea is to run or pedal or swim as fast as you can for a short time — between 10 and 20 seconds. Then catch your breath and do it all over again.

In every muscle, there are fast-twitch and slow-twitch fibers. While an individual's proportion of fast-twitch to slow-twitch fibers is largely determined by genetics — Olympic sprinters got there by choosing their parents well — you can increase your percentage of fast-twitch fibers somewhat with speed training. Your heart rate should go completely into the anaerobic zone, the place where your body pulls out all its energy trump cards. This corresponds to a reading of between 85 and 100 percent of your maximum heart rate.

---

## Failing to succeed

How hard should you be pushing yourself during a sprint? Harder. No, harder than that. No, even harder. Elite athletes do intervals until "failure." What does that mean exactly? It means that on your last set, you can barely stand up, or take one more stroke.

On a micro level, you have tried and you have failed. And on a macro level, you have most definitely succeeded.

---

# *Building a Workout Plan*

In order to maintain a consistent workout regimen, you need to get out your calendar. What follows is a 12-week training program, divided into three phases, that's guaranteed to get you in top shape in as little time as possible.

✔ Phase 1 of the program focuses on building an endurance base (see Table 1-2). You start out working out three days a week, all LSD workouts. By the end of this phase, you're exercising four days a week and are doing some strength workouts.

✔ Phase 2 of the program focuses on maintaining your endurance while building your power (see Table 1-3). You start out with one weight workout a week and increase it to two, while introducing some speed work by the end of phase two.

✔ Phase 3 of the program focuses on maintaining your strength and endurance, while adding some speed work (see Table 1-4).

| Table 1-2 | | Workout Plan: Phase 1 | | | | | |
|---|---|---|---|---|---|---|---|
| **Week** | **Sun** | **Mon** | **Tue** | **Wed** | **Thu** | **Fri** | **Sat** |
| 1 | 45 min LSD | Rest | Rest | 30 min LSD | Rest | Rest | 20 min LSD |
| 2 | 60 min LSD | Rest | Rest | 30 min LSD | Rest | Rest | 25 min LSD |

| Week | Sun | Mon | Tue | Wed | Thu | Fri | Sat |
|---|---|---|---|---|---|---|---|
| 3 | 60 min LSD | Rest | 20 min LSD | Rest | 30 min LSD | Rest | 30 min LSD |
| 4 | 75 min LSD | Rest | 30 min Strength | Rest | 30 min LSD | Rest | 30 min LSD |

**Table 1-3　　　　Workout Plan: Phase 2**

| Week | Sun | Mon | Tue | Wed | Thu | Fri | Sat |
|---|---|---|---|---|---|---|---|
| 5 | 75 min LSD | Rest | Rest | Strength | Rest | 40 min LSD | Rest |
| 6 | 90 min LSD | Rest | Rest | Strength | Rest | 40 min LSD | Rest |
| 7 | 100 min LSD | Rest | Strength | Rest | 40 min LSD | Rest | 30 min Strength |
| 8 | 100 min LSD | Rest | 30 min Speed | Rest | 50 min LSD | Rest | Strength |

**Table 1-4　　　　Workout Plan: Phase 3**

| Week | Sun | Mon | Tue | Wed | Thu | Fri | Sat |
|---|---|---|---|---|---|---|---|
| 9 | 30 min Strength | Rest | 30 min Speed | Rest | 40 min LSD | Rest | 110 min LSD |
| 10 | 40 min Strength | Rest | 30 min Speed | Rest | 40 min LSD | Rest | 110 min LSD |
| 11 | 40 min Strength | Rest | 40 min Speed | Rest | 50 min LSD | Rest | 110 min LSD |
| 12 | 50 min Strength | Rest | 40 min Speed | Rest | 50 min LSD | Rest | 110 min LSD |

What do you do when you reach week 12? Try the maintenance week schedule in Table 1-5 for a few weeks, which replaces one of the speed workouts with an LSD workout.

| Table 1-5 | | Workout Plan: Maintenance | | | | |
|---|---|---|---|---|---|---|
| **Sun** | **Mon** | **Tue** | **Wed** | **Thu** | **Fri** | **Sat** |
| 90 min LSD | Rest | 40 min Speed | Rest | 50 min LSD | Rest | 40 min Strength |

No, the program isn't carved in stone, and you can feel free to adapt this training plan to your schedule and your level of fitness. However, note that there are some overriding principles in any good training program:

- ✔ You should alternate weight lifting or speed workouts with LSD days or rest days to allow for recovery.

- ✔ Longer LSD workouts fall on a Saturday or a Sunday, which gives you more flexibility in scheduling them.

- ✔ Your aerobic output will increase from week to week, by no more than 25 percent a week during the endurance phase and no more than 15 percent a week during the power and speed phases.

# Chapter 2

# Just Warming Up

*A*lways be prepared. It's a good motto, even if you're not a Boy Scout. And prepared is exactly what you'll be, after reading this chapter. In these pages, you find out how to ensure that your workout will be, as the pharmaceutical companies say, safe, effective, and without unpleasant side effects.

In exercising, as in orienteering, a few minutes ahead of time spent getting yourself and your body prepared can pay big dividends down the road, making your workouts both more efficient and fun, as well as preventing injuries.

But unlike, say, getting your knot-tying merit badge, preparing properly for your workout is easy, if not always obvious. In this chapter, I discuss how to dress for comfort and efficiency, how to warm up and stretch effectively, and how to make the most of your workout time. So are you ready to get ready?

## *Bringing the Right Equipment*

One of the nice things about exercising is that for the most part, it's gear free. But just because you can go out and exercise with just what you can carry in a gym bag, doesn't mean that the right equipment won't make your life a little easier. Here's how.

## The right shoe on the right foot

A brief story about athletic shoes. A few years back, I went to my orthopedic surgeon with plantar fascitis — an inflammation of a tendon that made it feel like someone was plunging an ice pick into the bottom of my feet. First off, he did what any doctor would do: prescribe some anti-inflammatories to alleviate the pain and some stretching exercises to keep the tendon flexible. Then he asked me a question. "What kind of shoes are you wearing?"

"Whatever's on sale," I responded.

He said, "With feet like yours, you should be wearing Brand X or Brand Y. Brand Z is pretty wide, like your foot, but they're not going to give you the support that you need."

I did the math. I had saved $10 on the last pair of running shoes I bought. And I was paying the doctor $200 for 15 minutes of his time.

So I went out and bought a pair of Brand X shoes. Fit great. More importantly, within a week, the plantar fascitis was gone. And five years later, it's still gone. What more can you ask for?

 While I can't guarantee that picking the right footwear will keep the doctor away, I think there's a lesson here. Take some time to research the right footwear for your feet. Read magazine reviews. Check out the manufacturers' Web sites. Ask the advice of other athletes, and, yes, even your orthopedic surgeon. And once you find a brand and a model that works, stick with it. A shoe can't be a bargain if it comes complete with a trip to the doctor.

## Getting a brand-new bag

Do you have a gym bag? Great. Oh, you mean you don't? Then put down the book and go buy one, right now. Or soon anyway.

The right gym bag — and by that I mean one that's right for you — can make your life much easier. How? A sensible bag keeps your gear organized, which allows you to squeeze in a workout in a time slot where you once did nothing but scramble around looking for your tights and your lock.

What makes a good bag? One that's the right size — big enough to carry everything you need comfortably, but not so big that you're tempted to throw in the proverbial kitchen sink. Try to pick a style that you won't be ashamed to, say, carry to work.

The biggest practical need in a good bag is a way to segregate your wet clothes from your dry ones. The best bags have a partition, or a zippered compartment to keep the wet just-worked-out-in sweats away from the dry wearing-to-the-big-meeting clothes. Another big bonus is a breathable fabric — anything from Gore-Tex to mesh — which allows your work-out gear to dry without getting moldy. And smellwise, a bag that breathes will make you and your friends breathe easier, too.

# A Word About Workout Wear

Clothes may or may not make the man, but they *can* make your workout much more comfortable. And today's new generation of athletic wear is better than ever.

## Indoor clothes

The all-cotton T-shirt has long been a staple of the athletic wardrobe. And there are good reasons for it. It's cheap. It's comfortable. And it's easy to launder. But the problem is that it also absorbs sweat like the proverbial mop, which can make it less than comfortable after half an hour of hard exercise.

For those reasons, you may want to consign those Gap T-shirts to your casual wardrobe and get something a little more sports specific for your workouts.

New polyester and polyester-blend fibers don't absorb sweat as readily as cottons and they wick moisture from the skin to the exterior to where it can evaporate. Pretty cool, eh? That's exactly what you'll be if you give these new school threads a try. Pretty dry, too. Athletic clothes that do the wicking routine usually have a hang tag explaining how the gee-whiz fabric works.

## Outdoor clothes

If you're working out outside, you've got another set of obstacles to contend with — Mother Nature. And the problem, of course, is that the same clothing that keeps you warm can make you sweat enough that you get chilled anyway. But thanks in large part to man-made fibers, that has all changed. Here's what to look for:

- ✔ **High-performance polyester base layers** can wick moisture away from your skin so that the moisture evaporates before it makes you cold.

- ✔ **Fleece insulation layers** can keep you warm without bulk, and because they don't absorb moisture, they also won't get sweat-logged.

- ✔ **Breathable outer layers,** like shell jackets or pullovers, can protect you from the wind and rain (but not the gloom of night). The real trick is that these advanced fabrics, coupled with venting systems such as underarm zippers, allow enough air circulation that you not only stay dry from the inside but also from the outside.

# Warming Up to Warming Up

Do you have insurance on your house? On your car? Well, think of a good warm-up as insurance for your workout. Taking a few minutes before your workout to warm up can help prevent injuries and, yes, even boost your performance.

## The pre-stretch warm-up

When I hurt my knee a few years back, I went to physical therapy to rehab it, and each session was like a gym workout on steroids — figuratively, of course. And the first thing my physical therapist did every session was put me on the stationary bike for about 15 minutes. Then, and only then, did we start a thorough and lengthy stretching routine before we hit the weights.

Why, I asked. First, my therapist replied, contrary to popular opinion, stretching doesn't really warm up your muscles. What it takes to increase the circulation to the muscles and the connective tissue is some light aerobic exercise.

Secondly, serious stretching is important, but it isn't risk free. Overly enthusiastic stretching of cold muscles and joints is almost as likely to *cause* an injury as it is to prevent one.

And after filing this advice away, I began to notice this pre-stretching warm-up as one of the biggest differences between professional athletes and the rest of us. Watch recreational athletes, and the first thing they'll do is get down and start to stretch. But watch pros prepare for a game, and you'll find that the team trainers make them begin their workouts with a brief round of aerobic exercise, and only after they've begun to work up a sweat do they begin to stretch.

Here are some activities you can try to get the blood circulating, literally:

> ✔ **Pedal a stationary bike:** It's an easy, low-impact work-out that works your whole leg. Just remember to keep the RPMs high and the resistance very low.

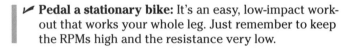

# Why tights?

Sure, there's something sexy about skin tight fabric over a trim body, but don't assume that its form-fitting cut is just for show. Recent studies have shown that tights made of Lycra or some other highly stretchy material can actually help to prevent muscle pain.

Essentially, the fabric exerts a mild compression on your leg muscles, which reduces the vibration that can cause muscle fatigue, as well as minimizes any inflammation if you overdo it. In short your tights are working the same way as a pair of support hose, or those burst-of-energy panty hose.

But don't overdo it. If your tights are too tight, it can constrict your circulation, and you could even injure yourself trying to wriggle inside. How tight is too tight? If it takes you longer to squirm into and out of your work-out clothes than it does to actually work out, that's a hint that you need the next larger size.

✓ **Take a light jog:** Again, it's important to hold yourself back. You're not doing aerobic work, you're just trying to increase your heart rate.

✓ **Take a walk:** No, it's not sexy, but a brisk walk is a good way to get the old blood circulating. And if you're really resourceful, you can combine it with transportation, walking to the gym or the beginning of your workout route.

If those ideas don't float your boat, just try something else to start the blood flowing. It doesn't really matter what you do as long as you keep the brakes on, so to speak, and don't go from breaking a sweat to working up a sweat.

## Protecting your skin

When you're exercising outside, it's important to protect your skin. Some simple preventive measures can not only reduce the risk of premature aging but also serious, and increasingly common, problems such as skin cancer. The following are a few common-sense suggestions on ways to keep from tanning your hide:

✓ **Use sunscreen:** Your first line of defense is a sports-specific sunscreen that won't rub off when you sweat or sting if it drips into your eyes. And make sure the SPF is at least 30. Apply it on all exposed skin whenever you're exercising outside. And, yes, that means even on overcast days, when 70 percent of the sun's damaging rays still get through.

✓ **Cover up:** While it's smart to consider your clothes a first line of defense against the sun, understand that a lot of workout wear isn't very high on the SPF scale. A white cotton T-shirt generally comes in at an SPF of 10 or less. So if you're exercising on a day when the sun is intense, or in a sun-intense environment such as when you're running on the beach, it's smart to apply sunscreen underneath your clothes.

# *The Power of Stretching*

For most of us, stretching has always been one of those things that you do because it's good for you — the athletic equivalent of eating your vegetables. And it's true that stretching prevents injury. But believe it or not, stretching can actually improve your performance, too.

Here's how it works. According to Dr. Vijay Vad, an orthopedic surgeon at New York's Hospital for Special Surgery, as you get older, the tendons that connect your muscles to your bones lose elasticity, kind of like a rubber band that's been left out in the sun too long. And as this happens, it restricts your ability to make the kind of explosive movements that you need to sprint or jump. (And, yes, this loss of the tensile properties in your tendons also makes you more susceptible to injury.)

The good news is that a program of slow, sustained stretching can actually restore much of the elasticity to your tendons, and in the process make you not only more limber, but more powerful, too. Here are a series of great upper- and lower-body stretches to get you started.

## A warm knee is a happy knee

Admit it. You like showing off your legs. Most athletes do. And while it does good things for your ego, it may not be doing good things for your joints.

Your knee, you see, is lubricated by something called synovial fluid. "If the knee joint gets cold, it makes the synovial fluid thicker," says a sports scientist with USA Cycling.

"Normally, it's the consistency of warm honey. When it gets cold out, it's like cold honey, and it doesn't work so well." How cold is cold? Well, most European coaches make their riders wear tights or leg warmers any time the temperature drops below 70°F. If you've got chronic knee problems, you may just want to do the same.

## *Lower body stretches*

In most exercises your legs are in constant motion. A stretching routine can not only increase your range of motion, and reduce the risk of muscle pulls, but can also prevent or alleviate overuse injuries like tendonitis. Of course, you can feel free to supplement these stretches with your own favorites.

✔ **Quad stretch:** Standing upright, and holding onto something for balance if necessary, bring the heel of one foot up to your butt and grab your ankle with your hand. Gently pull the ankle up until you feel a stretch in your quadriceps (the muscles on the front of your thigh). Hold that position for 30 seconds and repeat with the other leg. (See Figure 2-1.)

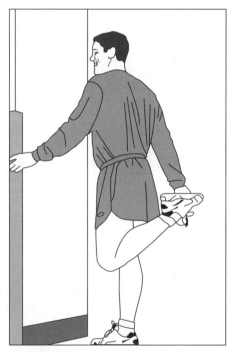

**Figure 2-1:** The quad stretch.

✔ **Hamstring stretch:** While sitting on the ground, extend one leg in front of you and bend the other leg, keeping the inside of your knee on the floor. Lean forward and grab the ankle of the extended leg. Don't curl your neck down, but try to move your chin toward your toes. You should feel a stretch in your hamstrings (the muscles on the backs of your thighs). Hold that position, without bouncing, for 30 seconds, and then repeat on the other leg.

✔ **A-stretch:** Stand with your feet spread about as far as they'll go. Slowly bend one knee until you feel a stretch on the inside of your non-bent leg. Hold for 30 seconds. Repeat with the other leg. (See Figure 2-2.)

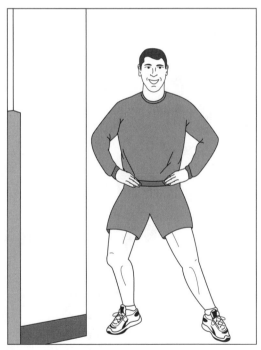

**Figure 2-2:** The A-stretch.

- ✔ **Calf stretch:** Step forward with your right foot as if doing a lunge. Bend your forward knee (keep your back leg straight) until you feel a stretch in the opposite calf. Hold that position for 30 seconds and then stretch the opposite leg. (Using a wall or some other object to lean against, you can stretch both calves at once, as in Figure 2-3).

- ✔ **Achilles stretch:** Stand with the balls of your feet on a step, but with your arches and heels dangling over. Hold onto a handrail for balance. Gently lower yourself until you feel a stretch in your Achilles tendons, just above the backs of your ankles. Hold that position for 30 seconds.

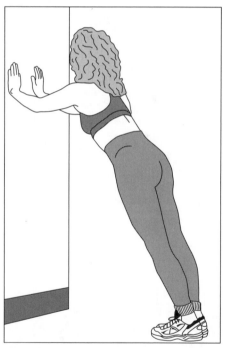

**Figure 2-3:** A double calf stretch.

# Upper body stretches

In most exercises, your upper body is especially subject to acute injury, from pulled muscles to more serious problems like ruptured discs and torn rotator cuffs. These stretches — along with any others you'd care to add — can help you reduce the risk of a trip to the doctor's office.

- ✔ **Hip stretch:** Lie flat on your back. Bend one leg up, grab your knee with both hands, and gently pull it toward your opposite shoulder. You should feel a stretch in your hips and buttocks. Hold the position for 30 seconds, again not bouncing. Repeat on the other leg.

- ✔ **Lower back stretch:** Lie flat on the floor, face down, with your legs straight and your arms extended. Pull your hands underneath you so that you raise your shoulders off the floor, but keep your hips on the ground. You should feel a stretch in your lower back. Hold for 30 seconds.

- ✔ **Upper back stretch:** Lie face-down with your legs extended and your hands next to your shoulders as if you were going to do a push-up. Move your hips off the floor, while keeping your knees and shins on the ground. Then move your hips back until your arms are fully extended, and you feel a stretch in your upper back between your shoulder blades. Hold for 30 seconds.

- ✔ **Shoulder stretch:** While standing with your back straight, reach across your torso with your right hand and grasp your left upper arm. Allow the left arm to bend. Slowly, pull the left arm until you feel a gentle stretch in that shoulder. Hold for 30 seconds, then reach with your left hand across your body and grab your right upper arm. Pull and stretch.

- ✔ **Forearm stretch:** Hold your right arm straight in front of you, extending from the shoulder and keeping your elbow straight. Raise your hand at the wrist, until your fingers are pointing straight up. The position is as though you were giving someone a stop sign. Hold for 15 seconds. Lower your hand until your fingers are pointing straight down. Hold for 15 seconds, then repeat the stretch with your left arm.

No pain/no gain does not apply to stretching. Stretching shouldn't hurt. If you reach the point of pain, you may be injuring yourself, so back off a little.

## Too sick to exercise? Maybe not . . .

You've got a lousy head cold, and, well, you're just not feeling like yourself. Should you bag your workout? It depends. If you're running a fever, or if you've got a hacking cough or significant chest congestion, you should wait until you get better. But if you've got the common cold, or a touch of the flu, you don't necessarily have to stay in bed.

Research has shown that light to moderate exercise can actually boost your immune system and help you fight off whatever's bugging you. The key, of course, is to make the workout mellow — a light jog is fine, but running dozens of wind sprints will probably just make you sicker. Just as important, help your body regulate its temperature. If the thermometer is below freezing, consider running on the treadmill instead of around the park. And when you're done, get out of those wet clothes so that you don't get chilled, which, old wives' tales to the contrary, won't make you sick, but can make you more sick by reducing your body's ability to fight off germs and viruses.

# Chapter 3

# Giving Yourself a Lift

● ● ● ● ● ● ● ● ● ● ● ● ● ● ● ● ● ● ● ● ● ● ● ● ● ● ● ● ● ● ● ● ● ● ● ● ● ● ● ● ● ● ●

*In This Chapter*

▶ Understanding the benefits of weight lifting

▶ Choosing your workout options

▶ Improving your form

▶ Staying safe in the weight room

● ● ● ● ● ● ● ● ● ● ● ● ● ● ● ● ● ● ● ● ● ● ● ● ● ● ● ● ● ● ● ● ● ● ● ● ● ● ● ● ● ● ●

Call it weight lifting, resistance training, body sculpting, or pumping iron, but whatever you call it, hitting the weight room is an increasingly important part of fitness.

Forget about the muscle-bound bodybuilders of yesteryear, preening in front of a mirror, and barely able to bend over to tie their shoes. Today's reality is that weight training can help anyone build a body that's not only aesthetic, but fully functional as well.

That's why it's a part of virtually every serious athlete's training regimen. A weight program can help you lose weight, play better, and prevent injuries.

In this chapter, I review the choices you will make while setting up a program. You discover how to save time without sacrificing fitness. I share some tips about improving your form to prevent injuries and maximizing your training benefits. And finally, you find out how to prevent accidents and injuries at the gym.

Because I can only offer a brief overview here, check out *Weight Training For Dummies* for more on the form, function, and benefits of weight lifting.

# The Benefits of Weight Lifting

Still not convinced? Then pull up a chair and listen in on some of the ways that weight lifting can improve your fitness, and, well, your life.

- ✔ **You'll look better:** Contrary to the myths about muscle-bound weightlifters, pumping iron is a great way to slim down. The theory is simple: Muscle is denser than fat. Increase your muscle mass, lose some fat (more about that in a moment), and, voila, you'll be able to fit into those slim-fit jeans sitting in the bottom of your pants drawer.

- ✔ **You'll lose weight:** Muscle burns more calories than fat. Adding muscle mass to your body therefore actually increases your metabolism, which means that your new muscular body is burning more calories 24 hours a day, 7 days a week. The bottom line is that if you eat the same amount of food and keep the rest of your daily activity the same, those calories are going to be consumed by newfound muscles, instead of becoming fat stores around your midsection, and you can lose weight where you would have gained it before.

- ✔ **You'll perform better:** Did you realize that 1932 Olympic 400-meter men's champion Buster Crabbe wouldn't have made the women's Olympic swimming *trials* in the same event for the 2000 Games? Or that Venus Williams serves harder than John McEnroe ever did? Is it evolution? No, genetic change doesn't happen over a few generations. The biggest difference between today's athletes and those of yesteryear is training, specifically weight training. In the first half of the century, most athletes did nothing more strenuous off the field than toss a medicine ball around. And as recently as 25 years ago, most world-class swimmers and tennis players had never even seen the inside of a weight room.

- ✔ **You can prevent injuries:** Done properly, a weight training program can actually prevent many sports-related injuries. Here's the logic: Most injuries affect some joint or another. Weight training can not only help to strengthen tendons and ligaments in the joint, but by strengthening the muscles around the joint, can help stabilize it and make those muscles less susceptible to strains, sprains, and general wear and tear.

# Making Your Choices

There's more than one way to lift a weight. And by making the right choices, you can tailor your weight training program to your needs and your lifestyle. Here's a quick primer, complete with the pros and cons behind each workout choice.

## Machines . . .

Every gym has them — a forest of big, shiny resistance machines that might have amazed Rube Goldberg. But are they right for you?

Pros:

- In large part, weight machines act as a mechanical strength-training coach. They pretty much guide you into doing an exercise correctly, especially if you follow the instructions printed on the side. And by following the recommended circuit, you get a solid full-body workout without much planning on your part.

- More advanced lifters like the fact that many machines are well designed to isolate hard-to-target muscle groups. And with most machines, it's impossible to drop a weight on yourself, so you don't need a spotter.

Cons:

- Few of us have the space or the money to put machines in our home gyms. And even at the health club, there's usually only one of each machine. Which means that, especially during peak hours, you'll often have to cool your heels while someone else is using the next machine on your circuit.

- And of course there's always the possibility that the club simply doesn't have the machine you want to use.

## . . . Or free weights?

If you grew up watching *Popeye*, you know about barbells and dumbbells. Do they deserve a place in your fitness routine?

Pros:

> ✓ Free weights are simple and inexpensive and remarkably versatile. With just a basic weight set and a bench you can do dozens, no, hundreds of different exercises. You can choose exactly the right weight for any individual exercise, by combining large and small plates.

> ✓ Because they demand that you balance and control the dumbbell or the barbell, free weights do a better job of mimicking the real world demand that sports — and life — place on your muscles.

Cons:

> ✓ Free weights do take a bit more skill to use. It's easier to "cheat" than with machines, and it's possible to injure yourself if you're not using proper form.

> ✓ If you're using heavy barbells, you need to employ a spotter to assist you in case you lose control of the weight.

## At home . . .

More and more fitness enthusiasts are finding that when it comes to working out, there's no place like home. Here are some of the benefits and drawbacks.

Pros:

> ✓ The good thing about home is that it's close. In the time that it takes you to get to a club, you can probably do a short, but intense, workout at home. And not have to worry about the commute home.

> ✓ Unlike a health club, your home gym is open at 6:00 a.m. or 12:30 at night or whenever you feel like — or can spare the time for — working out.

Cons:

> ✓ Of course, you have to devote a portion of your precious floor space to your gym setup. And most of us don't have room to put a full-fledged machine-equipped gym in our basement.

> ✔ If we did have the room, we probably wouldn't have the
>   money — $25,000 and up.

## . . . Or the gym?

The weights are there. The machines are there. A supply of
clean towels is even there. Going to a gym or health club is
still a standby for resistance training. But should you join?

Pros:

> ✔ There's a lot to be said for getting out of the house. You
>   leave the phone, the computer, the kids, and any other
>   distractions you can name behind.
>
> ✔ Gyms can also have a social element, whether it's
>   making small talk with a couple of buddies with the
>   same workout schedule or trying to find a date for next
>   Saturday night.

Cons:

> ✔ Gyms have memberships fees, and whether you're pony-
>   ing up month by month or on an annual basis, you're
>   paying whether you go to the gym or not, no matter how
>   good your excuse.
>
> ✔ And, of course, you have to factor your two-way com-
>   muting time into any do-I-have-time-to-work-out
>   equation.

## With a trainer . . .

Personal trainers aren't just for actresses and CEOs anymore.
Lots of ordinary people are finding it worthwhile to work out
with a specialist who can help them plan a program and stick
to it. Should you?

Pros:

> ✔ Motivation and results. If you can't get yourself psyched
>   up for a workout, your trainer will do it for you, either
>   through pep talks or the realization that you're paying
>   for the session whether you pump up or wimp out.

> ✓ More to the point, a personal trainer can help you focus your fitness goals, and work out a program that will help you reach them as quickly and efficiently as possible.

Cons:

> ✓ The biggest drawback to using a personal trainer is expense: They aren't cheap. Because the best ones are often in high demand, you sometimes have to adjust your schedule to theirs.
>
> ✓ And if the source of your motivation is largely external, then you can run into what Oprah might call a codependency problem.

## . . . Or on your own?

You don't have to be Benjamin Franklin, but a major part of fitness is self-sufficiency — it's your body and you'll take the credit (or blame) for how it looks. That's why so many lifters work out on their own. But is going solo for you?

Pros:

> ✓ Working out on your own gives you the ultimate in flexibility. You're the boss. You set your own schedule. You decide where to work out. You decide which exercises, how much weight, how many reps . . . in short, everything.
>
> ✓ For the price of even a handful of sessions, you can buy a year's membership to a gym, or even set up your own home gym. After all, what good is a resculpted body if you're too broke to afford new clothes to show it off.

Cons:

> ✓ Weightlifting is hardly a team sport, but it's possible to take self-sufficiency too far. When you're lifting at home, it can be hard to find solid workout advice, or even someone to spot for you.
>
> ✓ Can you say motivation? I knew you could. When you've got nobody but yourself to rely on, it can be easier to take a quick trip to the refrigerator than a longer trip to the gym.

# Saving Time at the Gym

"It takes too long." That's probably the number one reason that people give for skipping their workouts. But the reality is that doing a set of ten reps, slowly and with good form, still takes well under a minute. With that in mind, it's easy to speed up your workout by being more efficient when you don't actually have the bar in your hand. Here's how:

✔ **Stop dawdling:** Go to any gym and I guarantee you'll find a couple of people sitting at a machine or a weight bench. Not lifting. Just sitting. While it's okay to take a breather, you can speed up your workout, and get an additional cardiovascular benefit from moving quickly from one exercise to the next.

✔ **Plan your plates:** With a little bit of advanced planning you can spend more time lifting weights and less time fooling around with the plates on your dumbbells and barbells. What does that mean? Start out with the exercise that uses the lightest weights, add a couple more plates and graduate to a heavier exercise, and so on and so on, until the bar is full and you're doing your heaviest exercise.

✔ **Skip around:** There's no reason that you have to move from machine to machine like it's a buffet line. If the machine you want to use next is being used, move to another one. There's another advantage to breaking out of this routine — by moving some of the last exercises in your circuit earlier in your routine, you can go at them with more gusto, and maybe even increase your weight.

✔ **Split up:** If your weight routine is taking too long — or you're experiencing too much soreness on your rest days — consider splitting up the workout. Do upper body exercises one day, and lower body exercises the next. Especially if you've only got a limited window of opportunity — your lunch hour, or 45 minutes on the way to work — a split workout will give you enough time to do all the sets you need without eating up too much of your day.

## No pain, no gain? No way

Do you have to hurt in order to reap the benefits of weight lifting? Of course not. Pain is your body sending you a message that something's wrong. So if you experience a sharp, acute pain while you're doing an exercise, stop immediately. It's probably an indication that you're lifting too much weight or you're using bad form.

If you experience acute intense pain, especially if it's in a joint, in the hours or days after a workout, that's also a bad sign. Take some time off, use the RICE regimen explained in Chapter 4, and, if it persists, see a doctor.

However, it's important to make a distinction between pain and soreness. It's inevitable that you'll experience a little — or maybe even a lot of — soreness in the days after an intense lifting session, especially if you're just starting a weight training program or adding new exercises to your existing program. This soreness comes from lactic acid buildup and microtears in your muscles being rebuilt. You're literally feeling your muscles getting stronger, and this is the feeling that the "no pain, no gain" slogan refers to.

# Weight Room Do's and Don'ts

Sure, you can learn a lot just by watching your fellow lifters. But many of the things that make a workout successful are fairly subtle. If you want to get the most benefit of your time in the gym, follow a few of these basic rules.

✔ **DO stay quiet:** Sure, you've seen those weight lifting scenes in television shows filled with weights bouncing off the floor, clanging like a boiler room. But while those sound effects may make for good drama, they don't make for good form.

- As a rule, the quieter you are, the better your form. When you're using barbells, you're generally trying to move the weight straight up and down. Side-to-side movement causes the plates to clang together and is a sign that you may be slightly out of balance.

- With dumbbells, clanging them together during an exercise is a sign that you're not controlling the weight like you should. And when you're exercising on a machine, the plates shouldn't clang. Let them down gently, keeping control over the weight so that it just barely kisses the rest of the stack.

✔ **DON'T hold your breath:** Breathe in. Breathe out. You do that while you're reading, so why not when you're lifting weights? You don't have to grunt like a hippo with a stomachache, but focusing on your breathing — inhaling as you bring the weight down, exhaling as you bring it back up — can help you to improve your form.

✔ **DO get negative:** How can you squeeze out twice the training benefit of weight lifting in the same amount of time? Many weightlifters focus all their attention on the "up" portion of the lift, and then just let gravity or the mechanical resistance of the weight machine return the weight to its original position. The "down" portion of an exercise — weightlifters call it the "negative" — can be just as useful as the "up." The key to maximizing your weight workout is to lower the weight slowly — no, more slowly than that — which works a complementary set of muscles.

✔ **DON'T lock your joints:** Straighten your knee. Then straighten it a little more. That's called locking your joint. And in general, that's a bad thing. When you're doing squats or bicep curls, for example, there should always be a slight amount of bend in your joints. Keeping a small amount of flex in the joint prevents injuries that can come with hyperextending the joint. Secondly, it gives you a better workout, because your muscles, not your joints, are supporting the weight.

# Staying Safe at the Gym

The good thing about the gym is that you don't have to worry about external hazards like semi-trucks and angry Rottweilers. On the other hand, if you do get hurt, you've got nobody to blame but yourself. Here are a few tips to help you prevent injuries and accidents while you're working out.

✔ **Ask for advice:** If you're using a machine, or attempting an exercise that you've never done before, be sure to ask someone — a trainer, a club employee, or even another patron — how it works. While you may feel a little self-conscious asking what might seem like a silly question, think about how you'll feel if you get injured because you didn't ask.

✔ **Use proper form:** Anything worth doing is worth doing right, especially if you don't want to hurt yourself. It's easy to hurt yourself when using free weights, but you can even get injured when using a machine if you don't follow the directions.

✔ **Mind the pulleys:** While machines are safer than free weights, they're not injury proof. So follow the machine makers guidelines, which include keeping your hands and clothing away from moving parts, including the weight plates, and only changing weight settings when the weights are safely back in the stack.

✔ **Be careful:** The focus on safety doesn't wait until you've lifted the weight, or end after your last rep. So when you're carrying barbells or weight plates, hold them with two hands close to your body. When loading plates on a barbell, make sure the collars are fully locked. And when you're getting off a bench or machine, keep the weight under control until it's completely at rest.

✔ **Employ a spotter:** When you're working with barbells, especially in exercises like squats or bench presses, ask another lifter to spot you. They'll stand by and help you rack the weight safely if you lose control of it.

If you're spotting another lifter, they're most likely to need your help on the first rep — they bit off more than they could chew, weight-wise — and the last rep — muscle fatigue is catching up with them. So there's no time to be spacing out.

# Chapter 4

# Cooling Down and Fueling Up

*T*o paraphrase the novelist Dorothy Parker, I hate exercising, but I love having exercised. Okay, that's not quite true. While the act of exercising often involves significant discomfort, there are few things in this world that compare with the afterglow of having just completed a great workout.

But while it's tempting to kick back as soon as you're done sweating, resist the temptation. The truth is, the minute your last workout is over, the preparation for your next workout is beginning.

The good news is that a lot of that preparation is fun — it involves high-on-the-hit-parade activities like eating, drinking, resting, and gloating over your accomplishments.

In this chapter, I discuss how to cool down, eat right, replenish your fluids, and rest the right way.

# The Cool-Down

Did you ever watch the Kentucky Derby? Do the horses slam on the brakes as soon as they cross the finish line? Of course not. Well, you shouldn't either. After your workout, you need a few minutes to allow your body to make a smooth and gradual transition from exercise to rest.

You need to give your heart rate an opportunity to slow from its exercise-induced frenzy to a calmer, resting rate. A cool-down also gives your muscles the opportunity to flush out the lactic acid — the by-product of anaerobic exercise that's commonly known as liquid pain — that would otherwise make you oh-so-sore the next morning.

So how do you achieve this graceful progression from the sweating state to the post-sweating state? Simple. Just slow down. If you're doing an aerobic exercise, simply taper down your speed and resistance. If you're running, slow to a jog, and then to a walk. If you're swimming, slow down your stroke. If you're on a bicycle, shift down a gear or two and gradually pedal more slowly. Most exercise machines that you'll find in the gym — stair climbers, elliptical trainers, and stationary bikes — do this for you by building in a cool-down period at the end of each preprogrammed workout.

As a rule of thumb, five minutes is a good length of time for a cool-down, which is why most machines have this length of time pre-programmed. But listen to your body, too, and feel free to extend your cool-down time after a particularly intense workout session.

If you're doing resistance training, just shift to aerobic mode for a few minutes and jog, walk, or pedal for a few minutes to get your body in motion. A round of light post-workout stretching can also help your form.

# Resting to Get Stronger

Here's the news you've been waiting for: If you want to get fitter, it's just as important to rest well as it is to work out hard. Elite athletes know this. They understand that while they're resting, their bodies are recovering from the day's exertion. "Recovery is just as important as the workout," says Steve Johnson, an exercise physiologist with USA Cycling. "The purpose of the workout is to stress the body and let it repair itself. The benefit of the workout only happens after you've recovered."

That's why it can be smart to make a workout plan that allows for a couple of nonconsecutive days off during the week, especially after a particularly hard workout, and to restrict yourself to "active rest."

 What's active rest? It's not vegging out on the couch or surfing the Web. It's moderate activity of the kind that you'd do to warm up for or cool down from a workout:

- Do some gentle stretching.
- Take a walk.
- Shoot a few baskets.
- Mow the lawn.

Active rest is anything that gets you moving without really breaking a sweat. This keeps your muscles from getting stiff and helps get the blood circulating to the connective tissue in your hips, your knees, and your ankles. And as long as you take it easy, your body will be able to divert its energy reserves into helping repair the damage that yesterday's intense workout inflicted, and it will build stronger muscles in the process.

## The morning after

Do you ever feel the peak of your soreness two days after a workout? There's a good reason for this. While the muscle pain you feel the day after exercise is largely caused by the aforementioned lactic acid buildup, the soreness you feel a couple of days later is caused by microtears in your muscles being repaired.

In moderate amounts, this pain is your body telling you that it's getting stronger. If you're experiencing so much pain that it's affecting your next workout, then it should be a signal for you to cut back. That old saying, "no pain, no gain," is right, but only to a point.

# Refueling Your Body

You know the old saying, "You are what you eat." So do you really want to be a Big Mac, a large order of fries, and a chocolate shake the next time you hit the gym? When you're exercising, food isn't food, it's fuel. Which is why you need to think before you chew.

## Eating before your workout

This is a balancing act. You need to eat enough to give you enough energy for your workout, but not so much that you end up slowing yourself down. In practical terms, proper pre-exercise fueling is mostly a matter of monitoring not only *how much* you eat, but *what* you eat.

As you found out after you left the all-you-can-eat buffet at Enchilada World, some foods are more easily digested than others. Generally, this means focusing on easily-digested carbohydrates and keeping fats to a minimum. If you're working out in the morning, cereal or yogurt is a better bet than a triple cheese omelet with a side of sausage. (I found this one out the hard way on a particularly strenuous bicycle ride following a particularly indulgent brunch.) For lunch, smart fueling means bypassing the bacon double cheeseburger with a crème brûlée chaser and going for the pasta salad with the dressing on the side.

Why are foods that are okay when you're chilling out such a no-no when you're exercising? Chalk it up to evolution. Back in the days when your ancestors were being chased by saber-toothed tigers, they needed all the help they could get. So your body developed a response to this fight-or-flight situation. When you're running away from a woolly mammoth — or just pedaling up a big hill — your body funnels most of its resources to your muscles, postponing nonessential functions, like digestion. So eating easily digestible foods allows you to keep your muscles well fueled and keeps your stomach from rebelling. In short, you could say that it's about staying on the right side of the line between eating and being eaten.

## Eating during your workout

Should you eat during your workout? Probably not. If you're just going to the gym or for a short run, you can wait until you get home. But if you're running a half-marathon, or going on a 50-mile bike ride, you should plan for some on-the-go refueling. The key is to do it early, before your energy reserves run low, and in small amounts and in regular intervals so that it's easily digested.

No, I don't mean you should stop at the drive-through window. A couple of bites of an energy bar or a little bit of fruit is enough. And keep in mind, I'm defining eating in the broadest possible way — that is, taking in calories. So if you chug some fruit juice or a sports drink, as far as your body's concerned, that's eating.

What should you eat? From a nutritional standpoint, it should be mostly carbohydrates, with a little bit of fat to mellow out the blood-sugar spike that can come from too much sugar. There is a multi-million dollar industry trying to get you to choose energy bars and energy gels for your in-ride nutritional needs. They're generally easy to eat, and nutritionally, they've done most of the thinking for you. If you like the way they taste and they make you feel more like a triathlete, go right ahead. But they're not magic. You probably have some perfectly good energy foods in your kitchen cupboard, such as those in Table 4-1.

| Table 4-1 | | Food for Exercise | | |
|---|---|---|---|---|
| *Food* | *Calories* | *Carbohydrates* | *Fat* | *Protein* |
| 4 fig bars | 200 | 46 g | 0 g | 2 g |
| 3 Rice Krispie treats | 225 | 45 g | 4.5g | 1.5 g |
| 1 Milky Way Lite bar | 170 | 34 g | 5 g | 1 g |
| 1 Power Bar | 225 | 42 g | 2.5 g | 10 g |
| 2 bananas | 220 | 58 g | 0 g | 2 g |

## The bonk

Are you one of those people who hates to stop at a gas station? You'll run your car until it's almost at E, right at E, and even a little bit below E. Did you ever push it too far? Well, when your body runs out of fuel during the middle of a long workout — more than an hour — it's called *the bonk*. While it sounds kind of fun, the symptoms aren't: sudden, extreme weakness, often accompanied by lightheadedness, nausea, and/or severe hunger.

Fortunately, it only happens during endurance events — triathlons, 100-mile bike rides, and marathon runs — and the prevention is simple: Eat before you exercise. Eat small amounts frequently while you're on the road. And don't wait until you feel hungry. By then, it's probably too late.

A linguistic note: In French, the bonk is called *la fringale,* a word so euphonic that a fine French restaurant in San Francisco adopted it as its name. Funny how the French can make something so unpleasant sound romantic.

As you can see, there's not all that much difference between performance food and what your mother would dismiss as junk food. All have a good amount of carbohydrates and an acceptably low level of fat, and they can be eaten easily while you're running or riding. And if you stop to eat, your choices widen even further.

## *Eating after your workout*

As soon as you're done with your workout, head for the cupboard, and get some carbohydrates into your system. Energy bars or drinks, fruit, pretzels, just about anything will do. It's not the time for a full meal, but an important chance to replenish your energy reserves.

And the timing is important. For the first half-hour after your workout, your body is primed to replace the carbohydrates you used to power your muscles during your workout. Once that window of opportunity has passed, you simply can't top off your tank as effectively.

After a couple of hours, it's time for a full meal. Here's the time for that well-balanced diet with an eye toward your long-term energy needs. It's a good time to fuel up with protein — something lean, like a chicken breast, pork tenderloin, or piece of fish. Some veggies add fiber and all sorts of nutrients to the mix. Round out the meal with a small side of complex carbohydrates — a baked potato, a portion of pasta, or even just some bread. As for the fats, just keep it in perspective. In moderation, fats are a necessary part of a balanced diet. What that means is that while an occasional pat of butter or sprinkle of grated cheese won't hurt you, you should pass on the ribeye steak.

# The Hydration Quotient

Do you ever get home from a workout, and before you step into the shower, you step on the scale? "Three pounds lighter than this morning," you congratulate yourself. While it's certainly gratifying to watch those numbers go down, the reality is that you're probably a little less fat and a whole lot dehydrated.

There are a lot of reasons why water is the most important nutrient there is. Water — in the form of sweat — helps your body regulate its core temperature, and if you don't replenish your body's supply, it's like running your car with the radiator only half full. When you mix dehydration with exertion, the result can be heat exhaustion and even, rarely, heat stroke. In its more moderate forms, dehydration can cause muscle cramping and even make you more susceptible to muscle pulls.

So drink. Lots. In the hours before your workout, remember to drink a couple of nice large glasses of water. As long as you're sticking to water, it's almost impossible to drink to excess.

Drinking while you exercise is almost a Zen thing. You need to drink before you're thirsty. If you wait until you're thirsty, you're already dehydrated, and you're fighting a losing battle. Plan to drink at least four ounces every 15 minutes — more often if it's really hot — and you'll be fine.

And don't stop rehydrating after you exercise. In the hours after a workout, you'll still need to drink to rehydrate your body. It's also important to throw some electrolytes into the mix. Energy drinks help your body replenish these vital chemicals, but sensible eating — pretzels for sodium, a banana for potassium — can also do the job.

How can you tell if you're dehydrated? Well, if I may be so crude, simply look at the color of your urine. If it's clear, or almost clear, you're well hydrated. If it's dark yellow, hit the water fountain, now.

# *Are You Overtraining?*

There is such a thing as too much of a good thing. If you don't believe me, ask the third runner-up in a hot-dog-eating contest. The same goes for fitness. There's a fine line between building up and tearing down, and it's easy to veer onto the wrong side of it. How do you know if you're training too hard? Listen to your body. Do you feel chronically tired? Like you're constantly on the verge of getting sick? Are you having trouble sleeping?

Those admittedly vague symptoms can all be symptoms of overtraining, especially if you've increased the duration or intensity of your workouts in the past week or two. The best objective way to monitor your training is to check your resting heart rate before you get out of bed in the morning. If your exercise program is working, your resting heart rate should stay basically the same or even gradually drift slightly downward as your fitness increases. If you find that your resting heart rate is increasing, it's a sure sign that your body's under stress.

Fortunately, unlike the common cold, there's a cure for overtraining. Just take a day or two off, and when you go back to training, take it a little easier until your first-thing-in-the-morning heart rate settles back down.

# Dealing with Injuries

Injuries are a part of athletics. Despite all your careful preparation, eventually you'll suffer some kind of an injury. The key, of course, is to treat the injury aggressively so that you can return to action as soon as possible.

## Acute injuries

Ouch! That's the sign of an acute injury. One minute you're exercising and the next minute you're writhing in pain.

If you're experiencing severe pain, numbness, or restricted movement in a joint after a fall, see your doctor immediately to rule out a broken bone or a serious dislocation of the joint.

For less serious orthopedic injuries — such as mild sprains or bruises — follow the RICE regimen (**R**est, **I**ce, **C**ompression, **E**levation) outlined later in this chapter, and if the injury doesn't heal within a reasonable period of time, see your doctor anyway.

## Overuse injuries

Overuse injuries, on the other hand, tend to sneak up on you. You're a little sore one day, a little better the next, a little more sore the day after that. And then one day you wake up and you can't walk down the stairs.

To prevent overuse injuries, be smart and listen to your body. If you're training for an event, increase your workload gradually. If you're experiencing pain during or after exercise, take a few days off, or do some cross-training which will help you stay in shape without aggravating your injury. And if the pain is severe, or persists more than a few days, see your doctor.

## Treating injuries

The basic treatment for most joint and muscle injuries is pretty similar, regardless of the cause. The standard RICE regimen is the place to start:

✔ **R is for rest.** Stay off of it — that means no weight-bearing exercises. Some recent research suggests that gentle, range-of-motion exercise can speed healing — call this active rest.

✔ **I is for ice.** As soon as possible, put an ice pack on the affected area to keep down swelling and inflammation during the first 48 hours after an acute injury. Icing after exercise can help reduce pain and inflammation of an overuse injury.

✔ **C is for compression.** Wrap the joint to keep down the swelling and inflammation. In the case of an acute injury, it means not taking off a shoe or a glove or a pair of tights until you can get home to ice it. If it's an overuse injury, wrapping the area can provide support as well as help reduce pain and inflammation.

✔ **E is for elevation.** Raise the affected body part to keep the swelling down.

After checking with your doctor, you can augment the RICE regimen by taking a non-prescription-strength anti-inflammatory (such as Ibuprofen). Anti-inflammatories can not only ease the pain of injuries and muscle and joint soreness, but also, more importantly, they can actually help promote healing by reducing swelling.

# Part II
# The Weight Training Diary

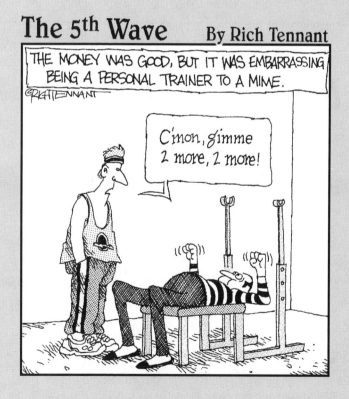

The 5th Wave    By Rich Tennant

THE MONEY WAS GOOD, BUT IT WAS EMBARRASSING BEING A PERSONAL TRAINER TO A MIME.

C'mon, gimme 2 more, 2 more!

## In this part . . .

Got your pen? Great. Because this is the part of the book that you write. The training diary pages in this section are your tabula rasa, a blank slate just waiting for you to record your goals, your accomplishments, and whatever else you'd like to put down on paper.

# Your Training Diary

● ● ● ● ● ● ● ● ● ● ● ● ● ● ● ● ● ● ● ● ● ● ● ● ● ● ● ● ● ● ● ● ● ● ● ● ● ● ● ●

*T*his is the part of the book that you write yourself, a customizable workout log where you can list your personal goals and record your progress. It's this section that makes this book truly your book.

At a minimum, you should record how long you worked out, how many reps at each weight you did in the weight room, or the duration and distance of your aerobic workout. You may also want to record how you felt when you got up and before, during, and after your workout.

Use this diary in a way that works best for you, but remember that I've assumed that you may not work out every day of every week — in fact, a good workout plan includes a healthy balance of exercise and rest.

- ✔ Track your progress over a ten-day stretch.

- ✔ Customize your journal each day for whatever workout you choose for that day.

- ✔ Write down your personal training goals in the, er, Training Goals section.

- ✔ Celebrate your training accomplishments in the Workout Wrap-Up section.

- ✔ Track your diet and nutrition goals in the Food for Thought section.

- ✔ And don't forget to note how you felt during your workout and what you should focus on for your next training session.

*"Do you want to get bigger and stronger? . . . Stop trying to make training complicated. Forget about this theory and that theory. Don't over-analyze the situation. Quit wasting time on arid intellectual debates. Leave the theorizing for the rest of the world. Go to the gym and train."*
— *Brooks D. Kubik, author of* Dinosaur Training

## Training Goals

Goals!

---

**Date:**

| Training | Time/Distance | Sets | Reps |
|----------|---------------|------|------|
|          |               |      |      |
|          |               |      |      |
|          |               |      |      |
|          |               |      |      |
|          |               |      |      |

### Food for Thought

---

**Date:**

| Training | Time/Distance | Sets | Reps |
|----------|---------------|------|------|
|          |               |      |      |
|          |               |      |      |
|          |               |      |      |
|          |               |      |      |
|          |               |      |      |

### Food for Thought

**Date:**

Training                    Time/Distance          Sets   Reps

_____

_____

_____

_____

_____

*Food for Thought*

_____

_____

_____

........................................................................................

**Date:**

Training                    Time/Distance          Sets   Reps

_____

_____

_____

_____

_____

*Food for Thought*

_____

_____

_____

........................................................................................

**Date:**

Training                    Time/Distance          Sets   Reps

_____

_____

_____

_____

_____

*Food for Thought*

_____

_____

_____

**Date:**

| Training | Time/Distance | Sets | Reps |
|----------|---------------|------|------|
| _____ | | | |
| _____ | | | |
| _____ | | | |
| _____ | | | |
| _____ | | | |

**Food for Thought**

_____

_____

_____

**Date:**

| Training | Time/Distance | Sets | Reps |
|----------|---------------|------|------|
| _____ | | | |
| _____ | | | |
| _____ | | | |
| _____ | | | |
| _____ | | | |

**Food for Thought**

_____

_____

_____

**Date:**

| Training | Time/Distance | Sets | Reps |
|----------|---------------|------|------|
| _____ | | | |
| _____ | | | |
| _____ | | | |
| _____ | | | |
| _____ | | | |

**Food for Thought**

_____

_____

_____

## Date:

| Training | Time/Distance | Sets | Reps |
|----------|---------------|------|------|
| | | | |
| | | | |
| | | | |
| | | | |
| | | | |

### Food for Thought

...........................................................................................................

## Date:

| Training | Time/Distance | Sets | Reps |
|----------|---------------|------|------|
| | | | |
| | | | |
| | | | |
| | | | |
| | | | |

### Food for Thought

### Workout Wrap-Up

| Accomplishments! | Notes |
|------------------|-------|
| | |
| | |
| | |
| | |
| | |
| | |
| | |
| | |

REMEMBER

*"Our most sacred convictions, the unchanging elements of our supreme values, are judgments of our muscles."*
— *Friedrich Nietzsche, philosopher and writer*

### Training Goals
Goals!

_____
_____
_____
_____
_____

..................................................................................

**Date:** [          ]

Training                          Time/Distance          Sets  Reps

_____
_____
_____
_____
_____

### Food for Thought

_____
_____
_____

..................................................................................

**Date:** [          ]

Training                          Time/Distance          Sets  Reps

_____
_____
_____
_____
_____

### Food for Thought

_____
_____
_____

**Date:**

| Training | Time/Distance | Sets | Reps |
|---|---|---|---|
| | | | |
| | | | |
| | | | |
| | | | |
| | | | |

*Food for Thought*

· · · · · · · · · · · · · · · · · · · · · · · · · · · · · · · · · · · · · · · · · · · · · · · · · · · · · · · · · · · · · · · · · · · · · · · · · · · · · · · · · ·

**Date:**

| Training | Time/Distance | Sets | Reps |
|---|---|---|---|
| | | | |
| | | | |
| | | | |
| | | | |
| | | | |

*Food for Thought*

· · · · · · · · · · · · · · · · · · · · · · · · · · · · · · · · · · · · · · · · · · · · · · · · · · · · · · · · · · · · · · · · · · · · · · · · · · · · · · · · · ·

**Date:**

| Training | Time/Distance | Sets | Reps |
|---|---|---|---|
| | | | |
| | | | |
| | | | |
| | | | |
| | | | |

*Food for Thought*

**Date:**

| Training | Time/Distance | Sets | Reps |
|----------|---------------|------|------|
| | | | |
| | | | |
| | | | |
| | | | |
| | | | |

**Food for Thought**

**Date:**

| Training | Time/Distance | Sets | Reps |
|----------|---------------|------|------|
| | | | |
| | | | |
| | | | |
| | | | |
| | | | |

**Food for Thought**

**Date:**

| Training | Time/Distance | Sets | Reps |
|----------|---------------|------|------|
| | | | |
| | | | |
| | | | |
| | | | |
| | | | |

**Food for Thought**

**Date:**

Training                                                Time/Distance        Sets   Reps

_____

_____

_____

_____

_____

### Food for Thought

_____

_____

_____

..................................................................................................

**Date:**

Training                                                Time/Distance        Sets   Reps

_____

_____

_____

_____

_____

### Food for Thought

_____

_____

_____

### Workout Wrap-Up

Accomplishments!                              Notes

_____          _____

_____          _____

_____          _____

_____          _____

_____          _____

_____          _____

_____          _____

## Training Goals

Goals!

_____
_____
_____
_____
_____

**Date:** _____

| Training | Time/Distance | Sets | Reps |
|----------|---------------|------|------|
| | | | |
| | | | |
| | | | |
| | | | |
| | | | |

### Food for Thought

_____
_____
_____

**Date:** _____

| Training | Time/Distance | Sets | Reps |
|----------|---------------|------|------|
| | | | |
| | | | |
| | | | |
| | | | |
| | | | |

### Food for Thought

_____
_____
_____

**Date:**

| Training | Time/Distance | Sets | Reps |
|----------|---------------|------|------|
| | | | |
| | | | |
| | | | |
| | | | |
| | | | |

*Food for Thought*

---

**Date:**

| Training | Time/Distance | Sets | Reps |
|----------|---------------|------|------|
| | | | |
| | | | |
| | | | |
| | | | |

*Food for Thought*

---

**Date:**

| Training | Time/Distance | Sets | Reps |
|----------|---------------|------|------|
| | | | |
| | | | |
| | | | |
| | | | |

*Food for Thought*

**Date:**

| Training | Time/Distance | Sets | Reps |
|----------|---------------|------|------|
| | | | |
| | | | |
| | | | |
| | | | |
| | | | |

**Food for Thought**

. . . . . . . . . . . . . . . . . . . . . . . . . . . . . . . . . . . . . . . . . . . . . . . . . . . . . . . . . . . . . . . . . . . . . . . . . . . . . . . . . . . . . . . . . . . . . .

**Date:**

| Training | Time/Distance | Sets | Reps |
|----------|---------------|------|------|
| | | | |
| | | | |
| | | | |
| | | | |
| | | | |

**Food for Thought**

. . . . . . . . . . . . . . . . . . . . . . . . . . . . . . . . . . . . . . . . . . . . . . . . . . . . . . . . . . . . . . . . . . . . . . . . . . . . . . . . . . . . . . . . . . . . . .

**Date:**

| Training | Time/Distance | Sets | Reps |
|----------|---------------|------|------|
| | | | |
| | | | |
| | | | |
| | | | |
| | | | |

**Food for Thought**

**Date:**

| Training | Time/Distance | Sets | Reps |
|---|---|---|---|
| | | | |
| | | | |
| | | | |
| | | | |
| | | | |

*Food for Thought*

........................................................................................

**Date:**

| Training | Time/Distance | Sets | Reps |
|---|---|---|---|
| | | | |
| | | | |
| | | | |
| | | | |
| | | | |

*Food for Thought*

*Workout Wrap-Up*

| Accomplishments! | Notes |
|---|---|
| | |
| | |
| | |
| | |
| | |
| | |
| | |

## Training Goals

Goals!

_____
_____
_____
_____
_____

**Date:** _____

| Training | Time/Distance | Sets | Reps |
|----------|---------------|------|------|
| | | | |
| | | | |
| | | | |
| | | | |
| | | | |

### Food for Thought
_____
_____
_____

**Date:** _____

| Training | Time/Distance | Sets | Reps |
|----------|---------------|------|------|
| | | | |
| | | | |
| | | | |
| | | | |
| | | | |

### Food for Thought
_____
_____
_____

**Date:**

Training                                Time/Distance        Sets  Reps

_____

_____

_____

_____

_____

**Food for Thought**

_____

_____

_____

........................................................................................

**Date:**

Training                                Time/Distance        Sets  Reps

_____

_____

_____

_____

_____

**Food for Thought**

_____

_____

_____

........................................................................................

**Date:**

Training                                Time/Distance        Sets  Reps

_____

_____

_____

_____

_____

**Food for Thought**

_____

_____

_____

**Date:**

| Training | Time/Distance | Sets | Reps |
|---|---|---|---|
| | | | |
| | | | |
| | | | |
| | | | |
| | | | |

*Food for Thought*

......................................................................................................

**Date:**

| Training | Time/Distance | Sets | Reps |
|---|---|---|---|
| | | | |
| | | | |
| | | | |
| | | | |
| | | | |

*Food for Thought*

......................................................................................................

**Date:**

| Training | Time/Distance | Sets | Reps |
|---|---|---|---|
| | | | |
| | | | |
| | | | |
| | | | |

*Food for Thought*

## Date:

| Training | Time/Distance | Sets | Reps |
|---|---|---|---|
| | | | |
| | | | |
| | | | |
| | | | |
| | | | |

### Food for Thought

_____

_____

_____

## Date:

| Training | Time/Distance | Sets | Reps |
|---|---|---|---|
| | | | |
| | | | |
| | | | |
| | | | |
| | | | |

### Food for Thought

_____

_____

_____

### Workout Wrap-Up

| Accomplishments! | Notes |
|---|---|
| | |
| | |
| | |
| | |
| | |
| | |
| | |
| | |

*"I believe that every human has a finite number of heartbeats. I don't intend to waste any of mine running around doing exercises."*
— Neil Armstrong, retired astronaut, first man on the moon

### Training Goals

Goals!

_____
_____
_____
_____
_____

**Date:** _____

| Training | Time/Distance | Sets | Reps |
|----------|---------------|------|------|
| _____ | _____ | ▢ | ▢ |
| _____ | _____ | ▢ | ▢ |
| _____ | _____ | ▢ | ▢ |
| _____ | _____ | ▢ | ▢ |
| _____ | _____ | ▢ | ▢ |

### Food for Thought

_____
_____
_____

**Date:** _____

| Training | Time/Distance | Sets | Reps |
|----------|---------------|------|------|
| _____ | _____ | ▢ | ▢ |
| _____ | _____ | ▢ | ▢ |
| _____ | _____ | ▢ | ▢ |
| _____ | _____ | ▢ | ▢ |
| _____ | _____ | ▢ | ▢ |

### Food for Thought

_____
_____
_____

**Date:**

| Training | Time/Distance | Sets | Reps |
|---|---|---|---|

**Food for Thought**

........................................................................................................

**Date:**

| Training | Time/Distance | Sets | Reps |
|---|---|---|---|

**Food for Thought**

........................................................................................................

**Date:**

| Training | Time/Distance | Sets | Reps |
|---|---|---|---|

**Food for Thought**

**Date:**

Training                                    Time/Distance          Sets   Reps

_____

_____

_____

_____

_____

*Food for Thought*

_____

_____

_____

---

**Date:**

Training                                    Time/Distance          Sets   Reps

_____

_____

_____

_____

_____

*Food for Thought*

_____

_____

_____

---

**Date:**

Training                                    Time/Distance          Sets   Reps

_____

_____

_____

_____

_____

*Food for Thought*

_____

_____

_____

## Date:

| Training | Time/Distance | Sets | Reps |
|----------|---------------|------|------|
|  |  |  |  |
|  |  |  |  |
|  |  |  |  |
|  |  |  |  |
|  |  |  |  |

### Food for Thought

..............................................................................

## Date:

| Training | Time/Distance | Sets | Reps |
|----------|---------------|------|------|
|  |  |  |  |
|  |  |  |  |
|  |  |  |  |
|  |  |  |  |
|  |  |  |  |

### Food for Thought

### Workout Wrap-Up

| Accomplishments! | Notes |
|------------------|-------|
|  |  |
|  |  |
|  |  |
|  |  |
|  |  |
|  |  |
|  |  |
|  |  |

*"We do not want in the United States a nation of spectators. We want a nation of participants in the vigorous life."*
— John F. Kennedy, 35th president of the United States

## Training Goals

Goals!

_____

_____

_____

_____

_____

**Date:** _____

| Training | Time/Distance | Sets | Reps |
|----------|---------------|------|------|
| _____ | _____ | | |
| _____ | _____ | | |
| _____ | _____ | | |
| _____ | _____ | | |
| _____ | _____ | | |

### Food for Thought

_____

_____

_____

**Date:** _____

| Training | Time/Distance | Sets | Reps |
|----------|---------------|------|------|
| _____ | _____ | | |
| _____ | _____ | | |
| _____ | _____ | | |
| _____ | _____ | | |
| _____ | _____ | | |

### Food for Thought

_____

_____

_____

**Date:**

| Training | Time/Distance | Sets | Reps |
|---|---|---|---|

**Food for Thought**

....................................................................................................

**Date:**

| Training | Time/Distance | Sets | Reps |
|---|---|---|---|

**Food for Thought**

....................................................................................................

**Date:**

| Training | Time/Distance | Sets | Reps |
|---|---|---|---|

**Food for Thought**

**Date:**

| Training | Time/Distance | Sets | Reps |
|----------|---------------|------|------|
|          |               |      |      |
|          |               |      |      |
|          |               |      |      |
|          |               |      |      |
|          |               |      |      |

*Food for Thought*

........................................................................

**Date:**

| Training | Time/Distance | Sets | Reps |
|----------|---------------|------|------|
|          |               |      |      |
|          |               |      |      |
|          |               |      |      |
|          |               |      |      |
|          |               |      |      |

*Food for Thought*

........................................................................

**Date:**

| Training | Time/Distance | Sets | Reps |
|----------|---------------|------|------|
|          |               |      |      |
|          |               |      |      |
|          |               |      |      |
|          |               |      |      |
|          |               |      |      |

*Food for Thought*

**Date:**

| Training | Time/Distance | Sets | Reps |
|---|---|---|---|
| | | | |
| | | | |
| | | | |
| | | | |
| | | | |

### Food for Thought

........................................................................................................

**Date:**

| Training | Time/Distance | Sets | Reps |
|---|---|---|---|
| | | | |
| | | | |
| | | | |
| | | | |
| | | | |

### Food for Thought

### Workout Wrap-Up

| Accomplishments! | Notes |
|---|---|
| | |
| | |
| | |
| | |
| | |
| | |
| | |

### Training Goals

Goals!

_____

_____

_____

_____

_____

....................................................................................

**Date:** [          ]

| Training | Time/Distance | Sets | Reps |
|----------|---------------|------|------|
| _____ | _____ | | |
| _____ | _____ | | |
| _____ | _____ | | |
| _____ | _____ | | |
| _____ | _____ | | |

### Food for Thought

_____

_____

_____

....................................................................................

**Date:** [          ]

| Training | Time/Distance | Sets | Reps |
|----------|---------------|------|------|
| _____ | _____ | | |
| _____ | _____ | | |
| _____ | _____ | | |
| _____ | _____ | | |
| _____ | _____ | | |

### Food for Thought

_____

_____

_____

**Date:**

| Training | Time/Distance | Sets | Reps |
|---|---|---|---|
| | | | |

### Food for Thought

---

**Date:**

| Training | Time/Distance | Sets | Reps |
|---|---|---|---|
| | | | |

### Food for Thought

---

**Date:**

| Training | Time/Distance | Sets | Reps |
|---|---|---|---|
| | | | |

### Food for Thought

**Date:**

Training | Time/Distance | Sets | Reps
--- | --- | --- | ---
 | | |
 | | |
 | | |
 | | |
 | | |

*Food for Thought*

---

**Date:**

Training | Time/Distance | Sets | Reps
--- | --- | --- | ---
 | | |
 | | |
 | | |
 | | |
 | | |

*Food for Thought*

---

**Date:**

Training | Time/Distance | Sets | Reps
--- | --- | --- | ---
 | | |
 | | |
 | | |
 | | |

*Food for Thought*

**Date:**

| Training | Time/Distance | Sets | Reps |
|---|---|---|---|
| | | | |
| | | | |
| | | | |
| | | | |
| | | | |

**Food for Thought**

...........................................................................................................................

**Date:**

| Training | Time/Distance | Sets | Reps |
|---|---|---|---|
| | | | |
| | | | |
| | | | |
| | | | |
| | | | |

**Food for Thought**

**Workout Wrap-Up**

| Accomplishments! | Notes |
|---|---|
| | |
| | |
| | |
| | |
| | |
| | |
| | |
| | |

*"It is almost impossible to be positive about training while being negative about most other aspects of your life."*
— David Whitsett, author of
The Non-Runners Marathon Trainer

### Training Goals
Goals!

_____
_____
_____
_____
_____

**Date:** [          ]

| Training | Time/Distance | Sets | Reps |
|----------|---------------|------|------|
| _____ | _____ | | |
| _____ | _____ | | |
| _____ | _____ | | |
| _____ | _____ | | |
| _____ | _____ | | |

### Food for Thought
_____
_____
_____

**Date:** [          ]

| Training | Time/Distance | Sets | Reps |
|----------|---------------|------|------|
| _____ | _____ | | |
| _____ | _____ | | |
| _____ | _____ | | |
| _____ | _____ | | |
| _____ | _____ | | |

### Food for Thought
_____
_____
_____

**Date:**

Training                                    Time/Distance          Sets    Reps

_____          ▢       ▢
_____          ▢       ▢
_____          ▢       ▢
_____          ▢       ▢
_____          ▢       ▢

*Food for Thought*

_____
_____
_____

. . . . . . . . . . . . . . . . . . . . . . . . . . . . . . . . . . . . . . . . . . . . . . . . . . . . . . . . . . . . . . . .

**Date:**

Training                                    Time/Distance          Sets    Reps

_____          ▢       ▢
_____          ▢       ▢
_____          ▢       ▢
_____          ▢       ▢
_____          ▢       ▢

*Food for Thought*

_____
_____
_____

. . . . . . . . . . . . . . . . . . . . . . . . . . . . . . . . . . . . . . . . . . . . . . . . . . . . . . . . . . . . . . . .

**Date:**

Training                                    Time/Distance          Sets    Reps

_____          ▢       ▢
_____          ▢       ▢
_____          ▢       ▢
_____          ▢       ▢
_____          ▢       ▢

*Food for Thought*

_____
_____
_____

**Date:**

| Training | Time/Distance | Sets | Reps |
|----------|---------------|------|------|
| | | | |

**Food for Thought**

---

**Date:**

| Training | Time/Distance | Sets | Reps |
|----------|---------------|------|------|
| | | | |

**Food for Thought**

---

**Date:**

| Training | Time/Distance | Sets | Reps |
|----------|---------------|------|------|
| | | | |

**Food for Thought**

**Date:**

| Training | Time/Distance | Sets | Reps |
|----------|---------------|------|------|
| | | | |
| | | | |
| | | | |
| | | | |
| | | | |

*Food for Thought*

........................................................................................................

**Date:**

| Training | Time/Distance | Sets | Reps |
|----------|---------------|------|------|
| | | | |
| | | | |
| | | | |
| | | | |
| | | | |

*Food for Thought*

*Workout Wrap-Up*

Accomplishments!                    Notes

*"The guy with the biggest butt lifts the biggest weights."*
— *Paul Anderson, Olympic champion weightlifter*

## Training Goals

Goals!

_____
_____
_____
_____
_____

**Date:** _____

| Training | Time/Distance | Sets | Reps |
|----------|---------------|------|------|
| _____ | _____ | | |
| _____ | _____ | | |
| _____ | _____ | | |
| _____ | _____ | | |
| _____ | _____ | | |

### Food for Thought

_____
_____
_____

**Date:** _____

| Training | Time/Distance | Sets | Reps |
|----------|---------------|------|------|
| _____ | _____ | | |
| _____ | _____ | | |
| _____ | _____ | | |
| _____ | _____ | | |
| _____ | _____ | | |

### Food for Thought

_____
_____
_____

**Date:**

Training            Time/Distance     Sets   Reps

_____

_____

_____

_____

_____

**Food for Thought**

_____

_____

_____

.......................................................................................

**Date:**

Training            Time/Distance     Sets   Reps

_____

_____

_____

_____

_____

**Food for Thought**

_____

_____

_____

.......................................................................................

**Date:**

Training            Time/Distance     Sets   Reps

_____

_____

_____

_____

_____

**Food for Thought**

_____

_____

_____

**Date:**

Training                                   Time/Distance        Sets   Reps

_____

_____

_____

_____

_____

### Food for Thought

_____

_____

_____

..................................................................................................

**Date:**

Training                                   Time/Distance        Sets   Reps

_____

_____

_____

_____

_____

### Food for Thought

_____

_____

_____

..................................................................................................

**Date:**

Training                                   Time/Distance        Sets   Reps

_____

_____

_____

_____

_____

### Food for Thought

_____

_____

_____

**Date:**

| Training | Time/Distance | Sets | Reps |
|---|---|---|---|
| | | | |
| | | | |
| | | | |
| | | | |
| | | | |

**Food for Thought**

..........................................................................................

**Date:**

| Training | Time/Distance | Sets | Reps |
|---|---|---|---|
| | | | |
| | | | |
| | | | |
| | | | |
| | | | |

**Food for Thought**

**Workout Wrap-Up**

| Accomplishments! | Notes |
|---|---|
| | |
| | |
| | |
| | |
| | |
| | |
| | |

*"Avoid running at all times. Don't look back. Something may be gaining on you."*

— Leroy "Satchel" Paige, Hall of Fame pitcher

## Training Goals

Goals!

_____

_____

_____

_____

_____

........................................................................................

### Date:

| Training | Time/Distance | Sets | Reps |
|---|---|---|---|
| | | | |
| | | | |
| | | | |
| | | | |
| | | | |

### Food for Thought

_____

_____

_____

........................................................................................

### Date:

| Training | Time/Distance | Sets | Reps |
|---|---|---|---|
| | | | |
| | | | |
| | | | |
| | | | |
| | | | |

### Food for Thought

_____

_____

_____

**Date:**

| Training | Time/Distance | Sets | Reps |
|---|---|---|---|
| | | | |
| | | | |
| | | | |
| | | | |
| | | | |

**Food for Thought**

. . . . . . . . . . . . . . . . . . . . . . . . . . . . . . . . . . . . . . . . . . . . . . . . . . . . . . . . . . . . . . . . . . . . . . . . . . . . . . . . . . . . . . . . . . .

**Date:**

| Training | Time/Distance | Sets | Reps |
|---|---|---|---|
| | | | |
| | | | |
| | | | |
| | | | |

**Food for Thought**

. . . . . . . . . . . . . . . . . . . . . . . . . . . . . . . . . . . . . . . . . . . . . . . . . . . . . . . . . . . . . . . . . . . . . . . . . . . . . . . . . . . . . . . . . . .

**Date:**

| Training | Time/Distance | Sets | Reps |
|---|---|---|---|
| | | | |
| | | | |
| | | | |
| | | | |

**Food for Thought**

**Date:**

| Training | Time/Distance | Sets | Reps |
|---|---|---|---|
| | | | |

### Food for Thought

........................................................................

**Date:**

| Training | Time/Distance | Sets | Reps |
|---|---|---|---|
| | | | |

### Food for Thought

........................................................................

**Date:**

| Training | Time/Distance | Sets | Reps |
|---|---|---|---|
| | | | |

### Food for Thought

**Date:**

| Training | Time/Distance | Sets | Reps |
|----------|---------------|------|------|
|          |               |      |      |
|          |               |      |      |
|          |               |      |      |
|          |               |      |      |
|          |               |      |      |

### Food for Thought

---

**Date:**

| Training | Time/Distance | Sets | Reps |
|----------|---------------|------|------|
|          |               |      |      |
|          |               |      |      |
|          |               |      |      |
|          |               |      |      |
|          |               |      |      |

### Food for Thought

---

### Workout Wrap-Up

| Accomplishments! | Notes |
|------------------|-------|
|                  |       |
|                  |       |
|                  |       |
|                  |       |
|                  |       |
|                  |       |
|                  |       |

*"He may win the race that runs by himself."*
— *Benjamin Franklin, writer and inventor*

## Training Goals

Goals!

_____
_____
_____
_____
_____

---

### Date:

| Training | Time/Distance | Sets | Reps |
|---|---|---|---|

_____
_____
_____
_____
_____

#### Food for Thought

_____
_____
_____

---

### Date:

| Training | Time/Distance | Sets | Reps |
|---|---|---|---|

_____
_____
_____
_____
_____

#### Food for Thought

_____
_____
_____

**Date:**

| Training | Time/Distance | Sets | Reps |
|---|---|---|---|
| | | | |
| | | | |
| | | | |
| | | | |
| | | | |

**Food for Thought**

---

**Date:**

| Training | Time/Distance | Sets | Reps |
|---|---|---|---|
| | | | |
| | | | |
| | | | |
| | | | |
| | | | |

**Food for Thought**

---

**Date:**

| Training | Time/Distance | Sets | Reps |
|---|---|---|---|
| | | | |
| | | | |
| | | | |
| | | | |
| | | | |

**Food for Thought**

**Date:**

| Training | Time/Distance | Sets | Reps |
|---|---|---|---|
| | | | |

**Food for Thought**

........................................................................................................

**Date:**

| Training | Time/Distance | Sets | Reps |
|---|---|---|---|
| | | | |

**Food for Thought**

........................................................................................................

**Date:**

| Training | Time/Distance | Sets | Reps |
|---|---|---|---|
| | | | |

**Food for Thought**

**Date:**

Training                                    Time/Distance          Sets    Reps

_____

_____

_____

_____

_____

*Food for Thought*

_____

_____

_____

**Date:**

Training                                    Time/Distance          Sets    Reps

_____

_____

_____

_____

*Food for Thought*

_____

_____

_____

*Workout Wrap-Up*

Accomplishments!                            Notes

_____         _____

_____         _____

_____         _____

_____         _____

_____         _____

_____         _____

_____         _____

_____         _____

*"There is a time to run and there is a time to rest. It is the true test of the runner to get them both right."*
— Noel Carroll, Irish Olympian

### Training Goals

Goals!

_____
_____
_____
_____
_____

---

**Date:** [          ]

Training                                    Time/Distance        Sets  Reps

_____
_____
_____
_____
_____

### Food for Thought

_____
_____
_____

---

**Date:** [          ]

Training                                    Time/Distance        Sets  Reps

_____
_____
_____
_____
_____

### Food for Thought

_____
_____
_____

**Date:**

Training                                    Time/Distance        Sets    Reps

_____

_____

_____

_____

_____

**Food for Thought**

_____

_____

_____

..............................................................................................

**Date:**

Training                                    Time/Distance        Sets    Reps

_____

_____

_____

_____

_____

**Food for Thought**

_____

_____

_____

..............................................................................................

**Date:**

Training                                    Time/Distance        Sets    Reps

_____

_____

_____

_____

_____

**Food for Thought**

_____

_____

_____

**Date:**

Training | Time/Distance | Sets | Reps
--- | --- | --- | ---
 | | |
 | | |
 | | |
 | | |
 | | |

*Food for Thought*

**Date:**

Training | Time/Distance | Sets | Reps
--- | --- | --- | ---
 | | |
 | | |
 | | |
 | | |

*Food for Thought*

**Date:**

Training | Time/Distance | Sets | Reps
--- | --- | --- | ---
 | | |
 | | |
 | | |
 | | |

*Food for Thought*

**Date:**

Training | Time/Distance | Sets | Reps
--- | --- | --- | ---
 | | |
 | | |
 | | |
 | | |
 | | |

**Food for Thought**

...................................................................................

**Date:**

Training | Time/Distance | Sets | Reps
--- | --- | --- | ---
 | | |
 | | |
 | | |
 | | |
 | | |

**Food for Thought**

**Workout Wrap-Up**

Accomplishments! | Notes
--- | ---
 |
 |
 |
 |
 |
 |
 |

### Training Goals
Goals!

_____
_____
_____
_____
_____

**Date:** [＿＿＿＿＿＿]

| Training | Time/Distance | Sets | Reps |
|---|---|---|---|
| | | | |
| | | | |
| | | | |
| | | | |
| | | | |

### Food for Thought
_____
_____
_____

**Date:** [＿＿＿＿＿＿]

| Training | Time/Distance | Sets | Reps |
|---|---|---|---|
| | | | |
| | | | |
| | | | |
| | | | |
| | | | |

### Food for Thought
_____
_____
_____

**Date:**

| Training | Time/Distance | Sets | Reps |
|----------|---------------|------|------|

### Food for Thought

........................................................................................

**Date:**

| Training | Time/Distance | Sets | Reps |
|----------|---------------|------|------|

### Food for Thought

........................................................................................

**Date:**

| Training | Time/Distance | Sets | Reps |
|----------|---------------|------|------|

### Food for Thought

**Date:**

Training                                    Time/Distance          Sets   Reps

_____

_____

_____

_____

_____

**Food for Thought**

_____

_____

_____

........................................................................................................

**Date:**

Training                                    Time/Distance          Sets   Reps

_____

_____

_____

_____

_____

**Food for Thought**

_____

_____

_____

........................................................................................................

**Date:**

Training                                    Time/Distance          Sets   Reps

_____

_____

_____

_____

_____

**Food for Thought**

_____

_____

_____

**Date:**

| Training | Time/Distance | Sets | Reps |
|----------|---------------|------|------|
|          |               |      |      |
|          |               |      |      |
|          |               |      |      |
|          |               |      |      |
|          |               |      |      |

### Food for Thought

_____

_____

_____

**Date:**

| Training | Time/Distance | Sets | Reps |
|----------|---------------|------|------|
|          |               |      |      |
|          |               |      |      |
|          |               |      |      |
|          |               |      |      |
|          |               |      |      |

### Food for Thought

_____

_____

_____

### Workout Wrap-Up

| Accomplishments! | Notes |
|------------------|-------|
|                  |       |
|                  |       |
|                  |       |
|                  |       |
|                  |       |
|                  |       |
|                  |       |

TIP

*"If a man coaches himself, then he has only himself to blame when he is beaten."*
— Roger Bannister, first man to break the four-minute mile

### Training Goals

Goals!

_____
_____
_____
_____
_____

........................................................................................

**Date:** [_____]

Training                              Time/Distance          Sets  Reps

_____
_____
_____
_____
_____

### Food for Thought

_____
_____
_____

........................................................................................

**Date:** [_____]

Training                              Time/Distance          Sets  Reps

_____
_____
_____
_____
_____

### Food for Thought

_____
_____
_____

**Date:**

| Training | Time/Distance | Sets | Reps |
|---|---|---|---|
| | | | |
| | | | |
| | | | |
| | | | |
| | | | |

*Food for Thought*

........................................................................................................

**Date:**

| Training | Time/Distance | Sets | Reps |
|---|---|---|---|
| | | | |
| | | | |
| | | | |
| | | | |
| | | | |

*Food for Thought*

........................................................................................................

**Date:**

| Training | Time/Distance | Sets | Reps |
|---|---|---|---|
| | | | |
| | | | |
| | | | |
| | | | |
| | | | |

*Food for Thought*

**Date:**

| Training | Time/Distance | Sets | Reps |
|---|---|---|---|
| | | | |

*Food for Thought*

........................................................................

**Date:**

| Training | Time/Distance | Sets | Reps |
|---|---|---|---|
| | | | |

*Food for Thought*

........................................................................

**Date:**

| Training | Time/Distance | Sets | Reps |
|---|---|---|---|
| | | | |

*Food for Thought*

**Date:**

| Training | Time/Distance | Sets | Reps |
|---|---|---|---|
| | | | |

*Food for Thought*

---

**Date:**

| Training | Time/Distance | Sets | Reps |
|---|---|---|---|
| | | | |

*Food for Thought*

---

*Workout Wrap-Up*

| Accomplishments! | Notes |
|---|---|
| | |

*"I cannot believe that our muscular vigor will ever be a super-fluity. Even if the day ever dawns in which it will not be needed for fighting the old heavy battles against Nature, it will always be needed to furnish the background of sanity, serenity and cheer-fulness to life, to give moral elasticity to our disposition, to round off the wiry edge of our fretfulness, and make us good humored and easy of approach."*

— William James, American philosopher

### Training Goals

Goals!

_____
_____
_____

........................................................................................................

| Date: |  |
| --- | --- |

| Training | Time/Distance | Sets | Reps |
| --- | --- | --- | --- |
| | | | |
| | | | |
| | | | |
| | | | |
| | | | |

### Food for Thought

_____
_____
_____

........................................................................................................

| Date: |  |
| --- | --- |

| Training | Time/Distance | Sets | Reps |
| --- | --- | --- | --- |
| | | | |
| | | | |
| | | | |
| | | | |
| | | | |

### Food for Thought

_____
_____
_____

**Date:**

Training | Time/Distance | Sets | Reps
--- | --- | --- | ---
 | | |
 | | |
 | | |
 | | |
 | | |

**Food for Thought**

........................................................................................

**Date:**

Training | Time/Distance | Sets | Reps
--- | --- | --- | ---
 | | |
 | | |
 | | |
 | | |
 | | |

**Food for Thought**

........................................................................................

**Date:**

Training | Time/Distance | Sets | Reps
--- | --- | --- | ---
 | | |
 | | |
 | | |
 | | |
 | | |

**Food for Thought**

**Date:**

| Training | Time/Distance | Sets | Reps |
|----------|---------------|------|------|
| | | | |
| | | | |
| | | | |
| | | | |
| | | | |

**Food for Thought**

---

**Date:**

| Training | Time/Distance | Sets | Reps |
|----------|---------------|------|------|
| | | | |
| | | | |
| | | | |
| | | | |

**Food for Thought**

---

**Date:**

| Training | Time/Distance | Sets | Reps |
|----------|---------------|------|------|
| | | | |
| | | | |
| | | | |
| | | | |
| | | | |

**Food for Thought**

**Date:**

| Training | Time/Distance | Sets | Reps |
|----------|---------------|------|------|
| | | | |
| | | | |
| | | | |
| | | | |
| | | | |

*Food for Thought*

...............................................................................................................

**Date:**

| Training | Time/Distance | Sets | Reps |
|----------|---------------|------|------|
| | | | |
| | | | |
| | | | |
| | | | |
| | | | |

*Food for Thought*

*Workout Wrap-Up*

Accomplishments!                    Notes

REMEMBER

"The function of muscle is to pull and not to push, except in the case of the genitals and the tongue."

— Leonardo da Vinci

## Training Goals

Goals!

_____

_____

_____

_____

**Date:** [                    ]

| Training | Time/Distance | Sets | Reps |
|----------|---------------|------|------|
| _____ | | | |
| _____ | | | |
| _____ | | | |
| _____ | | | |
| _____ | | | |

### Food for Thought

_____

_____

_____

**Date:** [                    ]

| Training | Time/Distance | Sets | Reps |
|----------|---------------|------|------|
| _____ | | | |
| _____ | | | |
| _____ | | | |
| _____ | | | |
| _____ | | | |

### Food for Thought

_____

_____

_____

**Date:**

| Training | Time/Distance | Sets | Reps |
|---|---|---|---|
| _____ | _____ | | |
| _____ | _____ | | |
| _____ | _____ | | |
| _____ | _____ | | |
| _____ | _____ | | |

*Food for Thought*

_____

_____

_____

**Date:**

| Training | Time/Distance | Sets | Reps |
|---|---|---|---|
| _____ | _____ | | |
| _____ | _____ | | |
| _____ | _____ | | |
| _____ | _____ | | |
| _____ | _____ | | |

*Food for Thought*

_____

_____

_____

**Date:**

| Training | Time/Distance | Sets | Reps |
|---|---|---|---|
| _____ | _____ | | |
| _____ | _____ | | |
| _____ | _____ | | |
| _____ | _____ | | |
| _____ | _____ | | |

*Food for Thought*

_____

_____

_____

**Date:**

| Training | Time/Distance | Sets | Reps |
|---|---|---|---|
| | | | |
| | | | |
| | | | |
| | | | |
| | | | |

**Food for Thought**

_____

_____

_____

**Date:**

| Training | Time/Distance | Sets | Reps |
|---|---|---|---|
| | | | |
| | | | |
| | | | |
| | | | |
| | | | |

**Food for Thought**

_____

_____

_____

**Date:**

| Training | Time/Distance | Sets | Reps |
|---|---|---|---|
| | | | |
| | | | |
| | | | |
| | | | |
| | | | |

**Food for Thought**

_____

_____

_____

**Date:**

| Training | Time/Distance | Sets | Reps |
|----------|---------------|------|------|
| | | | |
| | | | |
| | | | |
| | | | |
| | | | |

*Food for Thought*

........................................................................................................................

**Date:**

| Training | Time/Distance | Sets | Reps |
|----------|---------------|------|------|
| | | | |
| | | | |
| | | | |
| | | | |
| | | | |

*Food for Thought*

*Workout Wrap-Up*

Accomplishments!                    Notes

*"Exercise is bunk. If you are healthy, you don't need it; if you are sick, you shouldn't take it."*

— Henry Ford

## Training Goals

Goals!

_____
_____
_____
_____
_____

**Date:** [          ]

| Training | Time/Distance | Sets | Reps |
|----------|---------------|------|------|
| _____ | _____ | ▨ | ▨ |
| _____ | _____ | ▨ | ▨ |
| _____ | _____ | ▨ | ▨ |
| _____ | _____ | ▨ | ▨ |
| _____ | _____ | ▨ | ▨ |

### Food for Thought

_____
_____
_____

**Date:** [          ]

| Training | Time/Distance | Sets | Reps |
|----------|---------------|------|------|
| _____ | _____ | ▨ | ▨ |
| _____ | _____ | ▨ | ▨ |
| _____ | _____ | ▨ | ▨ |
| _____ | _____ | ▨ | ▨ |
| _____ | _____ | ▨ | ▨ |

### Food for Thought

_____
_____
_____

**Date:**

| Training | Time/Distance | Sets | Reps |
|---|---|---|---|
| | | | |
| | | | |
| | | | |
| | | | |
| | | | |

**Food for Thought**

---

**Date:**

| Training | Time/Distance | Sets | Reps |
|---|---|---|---|
| | | | |
| | | | |
| | | | |
| | | | |
| | | | |

**Food for Thought**

---

**Date:**

| Training | Time/Distance | Sets | Reps |
|---|---|---|---|
| | | | |
| | | | |
| | | | |
| | | | |
| | | | |

**Food for Thought**

**Date:**

| Training | Time/Distance | Sets | Reps |
|---|---|---|---|
| | | | |

### Food for Thought

---

**Date:**

| Training | Time/Distance | Sets | Reps |
|---|---|---|---|
| | | | |

### Food for Thought

---

**Date:**

| Training | Time/Distance | Sets | Reps |
|---|---|---|---|
| | | | |

### Food for Thought

**Date:**

| Training | Time/Distance | Sets | Reps |
|---|---|---|---|
| | | | |
| | | | |
| | | | |
| | | | |
| | | | |

### Food for Thought

..................................................................................................

**Date:**

| Training | Time/Distance | Sets | Reps |
|---|---|---|---|
| | | | |
| | | | |
| | | | |
| | | | |
| | | | |

### Food for Thought

### Workout Wrap-Up

| Accomplishments! | Notes |
|---|---|
| | |
| | |
| | |
| | |
| | |
| | |
| | |

*"Take care of your body with steadfast fidelity. The soul must see through these eyes alone, and if they are dim, the whole world is clouded."*

— J.W. Goethe, poet and dramatist

### Training Goals

Goals!

_____

_____

_____

_____

_____

........................................................................................

**Date:** _____

| Training | Time/Distance | Sets | Reps |
|---|---|---|---|
| _____ | _____ | | |
| _____ | _____ | | |
| _____ | _____ | | |
| _____ | _____ | | |
| _____ | _____ | | |

### Food for Thought

_____

_____

_____

........................................................................................

**Date:** _____

| Training | Time/Distance | Sets | Reps |
|---|---|---|---|
| _____ | _____ | | |
| _____ | _____ | | |
| _____ | _____ | | |
| _____ | _____ | | |
| _____ | _____ | | |

### Food for Thought

_____

_____

_____

**Date:**

Training                                    Time/Distance          Sets   Reps

_____

_____

_____

_____

_____

*Food for Thought*

_____

_____

_____

**Date:**

Training                                    Time/Distance          Sets   Reps

_____

_____

_____

_____

_____

*Food for Thought*

_____

_____

_____

**Date:**

Training                                    Time/Distance          Sets   Reps

_____

_____

_____

_____

_____

*Food for Thought*

_____

_____

_____

**Date:**

| Training | Time/Distance | Sets | Reps |
|---|---|---|---|
| | | | |

**Food for Thought**

........................................................................

**Date:**

| Training | Time/Distance | Sets | Reps |
|---|---|---|---|
| | | | |

**Food for Thought**

........................................................................

**Date:**

| Training | Time/Distance | Sets | Reps |
|---|---|---|---|
| | | | |

**Food for Thought**

**Date:**

| Training | Time/Distance | Sets | Reps |
|----------|---------------|------|------|
|          |               |      |      |

*Food for Thought*

....................................................................................................

**Date:**

| Training | Time/Distance | Sets | Reps |
|----------|---------------|------|------|
|          |               |      |      |

*Food for Thought*

*Workout Wrap-Up*

| Accomplishments! | Notes |
|------------------|-------|
|                  |       |

REMEMBER

*"The brain recalls just what the muscles grope for; no more, no less."*

— William Faulkner, Nobel Prize winner in Literature

### Training Goals

Goals!

_____

_____

_____

_____

_____

........................................................................................

### Date:

| Training | Time/Distance | Sets | Reps |
|----------|---------------|------|------|
| | | | |
| | | | |
| | | | |
| | | | |
| | | | |

### Food for Thought

_____

_____

_____

........................................................................................

### Date:

| Training | Time/Distance | Sets | Reps |
|----------|---------------|------|------|
| | | | |
| | | | |
| | | | |
| | | | |
| | | | |

### Food for Thought

_____

_____

_____

**Date:**

| Training | Time/Distance | Sets | Reps |
|---|---|---|---|
| | | | |

**Food for Thought**

· · · · · · · · · · · · · · · · · · · · · · · · · · · · · · · · · · · · · · · · · · · · · · · · · · · · · · · · · · · · ·

**Date:**

| Training | Time/Distance | Sets | Reps |
|---|---|---|---|
| | | | |

**Food for Thought**

· · · · · · · · · · · · · · · · · · · · · · · · · · · · · · · · · · · · · · · · · · · · · · · · · · · · · · · · · · · · ·

**Date:**

| Training | Time/Distance | Sets | Reps |
|---|---|---|---|
| | | | |

**Food for Thought**

**Date:**

| Training | Time/Distance | Sets | Reps |
|---|---|---|---|

### Food for Thought

........................................................................................

**Date:**

| Training | Time/Distance | Sets | Reps |
|---|---|---|---|

### Food for Thought

........................................................................................

**Date:**

| Training | Time/Distance | Sets | Reps |
|---|---|---|---|

### Food for Thought

## Date:

Training                                    Time/Distance        Sets   Reps

_____

_____

_____

_____

_____

### Food for Thought

_____

_____

_____

## Date:

Training                                    Time/Distance        Sets   Reps

_____

_____

_____

_____

_____

### Food for Thought

_____

_____

_____

### Workout Wrap-Up

Accomplishments!                            Notes

_____        _____

_____        _____

_____        _____

_____        _____

_____        _____

_____        _____

_____        _____

**REMEMBER**

*"Shall I show you the muscular training of a philosopher? What muscles are those? A will undisappointed; evils avoided; powers daily exercised; careful resolutions; unerring decisions."*

— *Epictetus*

### Training Goals

Goals!

_____

_____

_____

_____

_____

...................................................................

**Date:** _____

Training                          Time/Distance        Sets  Reps

_____            ▢    ▢

_____            ▢    ▢

_____            ▢    ▢

_____            ▢    ▢

_____            ▢    ▢

**Food for Thought**

_____

_____

_____

...................................................................

**Date:** _____

Training                          Time/Distance        Sets  Reps

_____            ▢    ▢

_____            ▢    ▢

_____            ▢    ▢

_____            ▢    ▢

_____            ▢    ▢

**Food for Thought**

_____

_____

_____

**Date:**

Training                                    Time/Distance          Sets   Reps

_____

_____

_____

_____

_____

### Food for Thought

_____

_____

_____

........................................................................................................

**Date:**

Training                                    Time/Distance          Sets   Reps

_____

_____

_____

_____

_____

### Food for Thought

_____

_____

_____

........................................................................................................

**Date:**

Training                                    Time/Distance          Sets   Reps

_____

_____

_____

_____

_____

### Food for Thought

_____

_____

_____

**Date:**

| Training | Time/Distance | Sets | Reps |
|----------|---------------|------|------|
| | | | |

**Food for Thought**

........................................................................................

**Date:**

| Training | Time/Distance | Sets | Reps |
|----------|---------------|------|------|
| | | | |

**Food for Thought**

........................................................................................

**Date:**

| Training | Time/Distance | Sets | Reps |
|----------|---------------|------|------|
| | | | |

**Food for Thought**

## Date:

| Training | Time/Distance | Sets | Reps |
|----------|---------------|------|------|
|          |               |      |      |
|          |               |      |      |
|          |               |      |      |
|          |               |      |      |
|          |               |      |      |

### Food for Thought

---

## Date:

| Training | Time/Distance | Sets | Reps |
|----------|---------------|------|------|
|          |               |      |      |
|          |               |      |      |
|          |               |      |      |
|          |               |      |      |
|          |               |      |      |

### Food for Thought

---

### Workout Wrap-Up

| Accomplishments! | Notes |
|------------------|-------|
|                  |       |
|                  |       |
|                  |       |
|                  |       |
|                  |       |
|                  |       |
|                  |       |

## Training Goals

Goals!

_____

_____

_____

_____

_____

---

**Date:** [ ]

| Training | Time/Distance | Sets | Reps |
|----------|---------------|------|------|
| | | | |

### Food for Thought

_____

_____

_____

---

**Date:** [ ]

| Training | Time/Distance | Sets | Reps |
|----------|---------------|------|------|
| | | | |

### Food for Thought

_____

_____

_____

**Date:**

Training                                    Time/Distance          Sets   Reps

_____

_____

_____

_____

_____

**Food for Thought**

_____

_____

_____

..........................................................................

**Date:**

Training                                    Time/Distance          Sets   Reps

_____

_____

_____

_____

_____

**Food for Thought**

_____

_____

_____

..........................................................................

**Date:**

Training                                    Time/Distance          Sets   Reps

_____

_____

_____

_____

_____

**Food for Thought**

_____

_____

_____

**Date:**

| Training | Time/Distance | Sets | Reps |
|---|---|---|---|
| | | | |
| | | | |
| | | | |
| | | | |
| | | | |

**Food for Thought**

---

**Date:**

| Training | Time/Distance | Sets | Reps |
|---|---|---|---|
| | | | |
| | | | |
| | | | |
| | | | |

**Food for Thought**

---

**Date:**

| Training | Time/Distance | Sets | Reps |
|---|---|---|---|
| | | | |
| | | | |
| | | | |
| | | | |

**Food for Thought**

## Date:

| Training | Time/Distance | Sets | Reps |
|----------|---------------|------|------|
| | | | |
| | | | |
| | | | |
| | | | |
| | | | |

### Food for Thought

---

## Date:

| Training | Time/Distance | Sets | Reps |
|----------|---------------|------|------|
| | | | |
| | | | |
| | | | |
| | | | |
| | | | |

### Food for Thought

---

### Workout Wrap-Up

| Accomplishments! | Notes |
|------------------|-------|
| | |
| | |
| | |
| | |
| | |
| | |
| | |

*"The secret of health for both mind and body is not to mourn for the past, not to worry about the future, or not to anticipate troubles, but to live the present moment wisely and earnestly."*
— Buddha, the Enlightened One

## Training Goals

Goals!

_____
_____
_____
_____
_____

---

**Date:** _____

| Training | Time/Distance | Sets | Reps |
|---|---|---|---|
| _____ | | | |
| _____ | | | |
| _____ | | | |
| _____ | | | |
| _____ | | | |

### Food for Thought

_____
_____
_____

---

**Date:** _____

| Training | Time/Distance | Sets | Reps |
|---|---|---|---|
| _____ | | | |
| _____ | | | |
| _____ | | | |
| _____ | | | |
| _____ | | | |

### Food for Thought

_____
_____
_____

**Date:**

| Training | Time/Distance | Sets | Reps |
|---|---|---|---|
| | | | |
| | | | |
| | | | |
| | | | |
| | | | |

**Food for Thought**

· · · · · · · · · · · · · · · · · · · · · · · · · · · · · · · · · · · · · · · · · · · · · · · · · · · · · · · · · · · · · · · · · · · · · · · · · · · · · · · · · · · · · ·

**Date:**

| Training | Time/Distance | Sets | Reps |
|---|---|---|---|
| | | | |
| | | | |
| | | | |
| | | | |
| | | | |

**Food for Thought**

· · · · · · · · · · · · · · · · · · · · · · · · · · · · · · · · · · · · · · · · · · · · · · · · · · · · · · · · · · · · · · · · · · · · · · · · · · · · · · · · · · · · · ·

**Date:**

| Training | Time/Distance | Sets | Reps |
|---|---|---|---|
| | | | |
| | | | |
| | | | |
| | | | |
| | | | |

**Food for Thought**

**Date:**

| Training | Time/Distance | Sets | Reps |
|----------|---------------|------|------|
| | | | |
| | | | |
| | | | |
| | | | |
| | | | |

*Food for Thought*

_____

_____

_____

**Date:**

| Training | Time/Distance | Sets | Reps |
|----------|---------------|------|------|
| | | | |
| | | | |
| | | | |
| | | | |
| | | | |

*Food for Thought*

_____

_____

_____

**Date:**

| Training | Time/Distance | Sets | Reps |
|----------|---------------|------|------|
| | | | |
| | | | |
| | | | |
| | | | |
| | | | |

*Food for Thought*

_____

_____

_____

**Date:**

| Training | Time/Distance | Sets | Reps |
|----------|---------------|------|------|
| | | | |
| | | | |
| | | | |
| | | | |
| | | | |

*Food for Thought*

.........................................................................................................

**Date:**

| Training | Time/Distance | Sets | Reps |
|----------|---------------|------|------|
| | | | |
| | | | |
| | | | |
| | | | |
| | | | |

*Food for Thought*

*Workout Wrap-Up*

| Accomplishments! | Notes |
|------------------|-------|
| | |
| | |
| | |
| | |
| | |
| | |
| | |

### Training Goals

Goals!

_____

_____

_____

_____

_____

........................................................................................

**Date:**

| Training | Time/Distance | Sets | Reps |
|----------|---------------|------|------|
| _____ | _____ | ☐ | ☐ |
| _____ | _____ | ☐ | ☐ |
| _____ | _____ | ☐ | ☐ |
| _____ | _____ | ☐ | ☐ |
| _____ | _____ | ☐ | ☐ |

### Food for Thought

_____

_____

_____

........................................................................................

**Date:**

| Training | Time/Distance | Sets | Reps |
|----------|---------------|------|------|
| _____ | _____ | ☐ | ☐ |
| _____ | _____ | ☐ | ☐ |
| _____ | _____ | ☐ | ☐ |
| _____ | _____ | ☐ | ☐ |
| _____ | _____ | ☐ | ☐ |

### Food for Thought

_____

_____

_____

**Date:**

| Training | Time/Distance | Sets | Reps |
|---|---|---|---|
| | | | |
| | | | |
| | | | |
| | | | |
| | | | |

*Food for Thought*

............................................................................................

**Date:**

| Training | Time/Distance | Sets | Reps |
|---|---|---|---|
| | | | |
| | | | |
| | | | |
| | | | |
| | | | |

*Food for Thought*

............................................................................................

**Date:**

| Training | Time/Distance | Sets | Reps |
|---|---|---|---|
| | | | |
| | | | |
| | | | |
| | | | |
| | | | |

*Food for Thought*

**Date:**

Training | Time/Distance | Sets | Reps
--- | --- | --- | ---
_____ | _____ | | 
_____ | _____ | | 
_____ | _____ | | 
_____ | _____ | | 
_____ | _____ | | 

*Food for Thought*

_____
_____
_____

. . . . . . . . . . . . . . . . . . . . . . . . . . . . . . . . . . . . . . . . . . . . . . . . . . . . . . . . . . . . . . . .

**Date:**

Training | Time/Distance | Sets | Reps
--- | --- | --- | ---
_____ | _____ | | 
_____ | _____ | | 
_____ | _____ | | 
_____ | _____ | | 
_____ | _____ | | 

*Food for Thought*

_____
_____
_____

. . . . . . . . . . . . . . . . . . . . . . . . . . . . . . . . . . . . . . . . . . . . . . . . . . . . . . . . . . . . . . . .

**Date:**

Training | Time/Distance | Sets | Reps
--- | --- | --- | ---
_____ | _____ | | 
_____ | _____ | | 
_____ | _____ | | 
_____ | _____ | | 
_____ | _____ | | 

*Food for Thought*

_____
_____
_____

**Date:**

Training                                    Time/Distance              Sets  Reps

_____

_____

_____

_____

_____

**Food for Thought**

_____

_____

_____

........................................................................................................

**Date:**

Training                                    Time/Distance              Sets  Reps

_____

_____

_____

_____

_____

**Food for Thought**

_____

_____

_____

**Workout Wrap-Up**

Accomplishments!                            Notes

_____          _____

_____          _____

_____          _____

_____          _____

_____          _____

_____          _____

_____          _____

_____          _____

REMEMBER

""The sovereign invigorator of the body is exercise, and of all the exercises walking is the best."
— Thomas Jefferson, American statesman and 3rd president of the United States

## Training Goals

Goals!

_____
_____
_____
_____
_____

....................................................................................................

**Date:** [_____]

| Training | Time/Distance | Sets | Reps |
|----------|---------------|------|------|
| _____ | _____ | | |
| _____ | _____ | | |
| _____ | _____ | | |
| _____ | _____ | | |
| _____ | _____ | | |

### Food for Thought

_____
_____
_____

....................................................................................................

**Date:** [_____]

| Training | Time/Distance | Sets | Reps |
|----------|---------------|------|------|
| _____ | _____ | | |
| _____ | _____ | | |
| _____ | _____ | | |
| _____ | _____ | | |
| _____ | _____ | | |

### Food for Thought

_____
_____
_____

**Date:**

Training                                      Time/Distance          Sets  Reps

_____

_____

_____

_____

_____

**Food for Thought**

_____

_____

_____

...................................................................................................

**Date:**

Training                                      Time/Distance          Sets  Reps

_____

_____

_____

_____

_____

**Food for Thought**

_____

_____

_____

...................................................................................................

**Date:**

Training                                      Time/Distance          Sets  Reps

_____

_____

_____

_____

_____

**Food for Thought**

_____

_____

_____

**Date:**

| Training | Time/Distance | Sets | Reps |
|---|---|---|---|
| _____ | | | |
| _____ | | | |
| _____ | | | |
| _____ | | | |
| _____ | | | |

*Food for Thought*

_____

_____

_____

..................................................................................

**Date:**

| Training | Time/Distance | Sets | Reps |
|---|---|---|---|
| _____ | | | |
| _____ | | | |
| _____ | | | |
| _____ | | | |
| _____ | | | |

*Food for Thought*

_____

_____

_____

..................................................................................

**Date:**

| Training | Time/Distance | Sets | Reps |
|---|---|---|---|
| _____ | | | |
| _____ | | | |
| _____ | | | |
| _____ | | | |
| _____ | | | |

*Food for Thought*

_____

_____

_____

**Date:**

Training                                          Time/Distance          Sets   Reps

_____

_____

_____

_____

**Food for Thought**

_____

_____

_____

..............................................................................................

**Date:**

Training                                          Time/Distance          Sets   Reps

_____

_____

_____

_____

**Food for Thought**

_____

_____

_____

**Workout Wrap-Up**

Accomplishments!                                  Notes

_____      _____

_____      _____

_____      _____

_____      _____

_____      _____

_____      _____

_____      _____

REMEMBER

"People say I've given people courage. That makes me feel good, but I don't see how I do that. I think my running is a selfish thing. But it provides the challenge that allows me to feel good about myself. How can I expect to do well in other activities if I don't feel good about myself?"
— Joan Benoit, Olympic Marathon champion

## Training Goals

Goals!

_____
_____
_____
_____
_____

### Date:

| Training | Time/Distance | Sets | Reps |
|----------|---------------|------|------|
| _____ | _____ | | |
| _____ | _____ | | |
| _____ | _____ | | |
| _____ | _____ | | |
| _____ | _____ | | |

### Food for Thought

_____
_____
_____

### Date:

| Training | Time/Distance | Sets | Reps |
|----------|---------------|------|------|
| _____ | _____ | | |
| _____ | _____ | | |
| _____ | _____ | | |
| _____ | _____ | | |
| _____ | _____ | | |

### Food for Thought

_____
_____
_____

**Date:**

| Training | Time/Distance | Sets | Reps |
|----------|---------------|------|------|
| _____ | | | |
| _____ | | | |
| _____ | | | |
| _____ | | | |
| _____ | | | |

**Food for Thought**

_____

_____

_____

---

**Date:**

| Training | Time/Distance | Sets | Reps |
|----------|---------------|------|------|
| _____ | | | |
| _____ | | | |
| _____ | | | |
| _____ | | | |

**Food for Thought**

_____

_____

_____

---

**Date:**

| Training | Time/Distance | Sets | Reps |
|----------|---------------|------|------|
| _____ | | | |
| _____ | | | |
| _____ | | | |
| _____ | | | |

**Food for Thought**

_____

_____

_____

**Date:**

| Training | Time/Distance | Sets | Reps |
|----------|---------------|------|------|
| _____ | _____ | | |
| _____ | _____ | | |
| _____ | _____ | | |
| _____ | _____ | | |
| _____ | _____ | | |

*Food for Thought*

_____

_____

_____

**Date:**

| Training | Time/Distance | Sets | Reps |
|----------|---------------|------|------|
| _____ | _____ | | |
| _____ | _____ | | |
| _____ | _____ | | |
| _____ | _____ | | |
| _____ | _____ | | |

*Food for Thought*

_____

_____

_____

**Date:**

| Training | Time/Distance | Sets | Reps |
|----------|---------------|------|------|
| _____ | _____ | | |
| _____ | _____ | | |
| _____ | _____ | | |
| _____ | _____ | | |
| _____ | _____ | | |

*Food for Thought*

_____

_____

_____

**Date:**

Training                                    Time/Distance          Sets   Reps

_____

_____

_____

_____

_____

*Food for Thought*

_____

_____

_____

**Date:**

Training                                    Time/Distance          Sets   Reps

_____

_____

_____

_____

_____

*Food for Thought*

_____

_____

_____

*Workout Wrap-Up*

Accomplishments!                            Notes

_____        _____

_____        _____

_____        _____

_____        _____

_____        _____

_____        _____

_____        _____

*"A pint of sweat saves a gallon of blood."*
— George Patton, U.S. Army General

## Training Goals

Goals!

_____
_____
_____
_____
_____

**Date:**

| Training | Time/Distance | Sets | Reps |
|----------|---------------|------|------|
| _____ | _____ | | |
| _____ | | | |
| _____ | | | |
| _____ | | | |
| _____ | | | |

### Food for Thought

_____
_____
_____

**Date:**

| Training | Time/Distance | Sets | Reps |
|----------|---------------|------|------|
| _____ | _____ | | |
| _____ | | | |
| _____ | | | |
| _____ | | | |
| _____ | | | |

### Food for Thought

_____
_____
_____

**Date:**

| Training | Time/Distance | Sets | Reps |
|----------|---------------|------|------|
| | | | |
| | | | |
| | | | |
| | | | |
| | | | |

**Food for Thought**

........................................................................

**Date:**

| Training | Time/Distance | Sets | Reps |
|----------|---------------|------|------|
| | | | |
| | | | |
| | | | |
| | | | |
| | | | |

**Food for Thought**

........................................................................

**Date:**

| Training | Time/Distance | Sets | Reps |
|----------|---------------|------|------|
| | | | |
| | | | |
| | | | |
| | | | |
| | | | |

**Food for Thought**

**Date:**

| Training | Time/Distance | Sets | Reps |
|----------|---------------|------|------|
| | | | |
| | | | |
| | | | |
| | | | |
| | | | |

**Food for Thought**

**Date:**

| Training | Time/Distance | Sets | Reps |
|----------|---------------|------|------|
| | | | |
| | | | |
| | | | |
| | | | |
| | | | |

**Food for Thought**

**Date:**

| Training | Time/Distance | Sets | Reps |
|----------|---------------|------|------|
| | | | |
| | | | |
| | | | |
| | | | |
| | | | |

**Food for Thought**

**Date:**

| Training | Time/Distance | Sets | Reps |
|----------|---------------|------|------|
| | | | |
| | | | |
| | | | |
| | | | |
| | | | |

**Food for Thought**

........................................................................................

**Date:**

| Training | Time/Distance | Sets | Reps |
|----------|---------------|------|------|
| | | | |
| | | | |
| | | | |
| | | | |
| | | | |

**Food for Thought**

**Workout Wrap-Up**

Accomplishments!                    Notes

*"Slow running just makes you a slow runner."*
*— Grete Waitz, nine-time winner of the*
*New York City Marathon*

## *Training Goals*
Goals!

_____
_____
_____
_____
_____

........................................................................

### *Date:*

| Training | Time/Distance | Sets | Reps |
|----------|---------------|------|------|
| _____ | _____ | | |
| _____ | _____ | | |
| _____ | _____ | | |
| _____ | _____ | | |
| _____ | _____ | | |

### *Food for Thought*

_____
_____
_____

........................................................................

### *Date:*

| Training | Time/Distance | Sets | Reps |
|----------|---------------|------|------|
| _____ | _____ | | |
| _____ | _____ | | |
| _____ | _____ | | |
| _____ | _____ | | |
| _____ | _____ | | |

### *Food for Thought*

_____
_____
_____

**Date:**

| Training | Time/Distance | Sets | Reps |
|----------|---------------|------|------|
| | | | |
| | | | |
| | | | |
| | | | |
| | | | |

**Food for Thought**

........................................................................................

**Date:**

| Training | Time/Distance | Sets | Reps |
|----------|---------------|------|------|
| | | | |
| | | | |
| | | | |
| | | | |
| | | | |

**Food for Thought**

........................................................................................

**Date:**

| Training | Time/Distance | Sets | Reps |
|----------|---------------|------|------|
| | | | |
| | | | |
| | | | |
| | | | |
| | | | |

**Food for Thought**

**Date:**

| Training | Time/Distance | Sets | Reps |
|---|---|---|---|
| | | | |
| | | | |
| | | | |
| | | | |
| | | | |

**Food for Thought**

_____

_____

_____

...........................................................................

**Date:**

| Training | Time/Distance | Sets | Reps |
|---|---|---|---|
| | | | |
| | | | |
| | | | |
| | | | |
| | | | |

**Food for Thought**

_____

_____

_____

...........................................................................

**Date:**

| Training | Time/Distance | Sets | Reps |
|---|---|---|---|
| | | | |
| | | | |
| | | | |
| | | | |
| | | | |

**Food for Thought**

_____

_____

_____

**Date:**

| Training | Time/Distance | Sets | Reps |
|---|---|---|---|
| | | | |
| | | | |
| | | | |
| | | | |
| | | | |

### Food for Thought

......................................................................................

**Date:**

| Training | Time/Distance | Sets | Reps |
|---|---|---|---|
| | | | |
| | | | |
| | | | |
| | | | |
| | | | |

### Food for Thought

### Workout Wrap-Up

| Accomplishments! | Notes |
|---|---|
| | |
| | |
| | |
| | |
| | |
| | |

*"Now my task is smoothly done/I can fly or I can run."*
— *John Milton, writer*

## Training Goals

Goals!

_____
_____
_____
_____
_____

---

**Date:** _____

| Training | Time/Distance | Sets | Reps |
|----------|---------------|------|------|
| _____ | | | |
| _____ | | | |
| _____ | | | |
| _____ | | | |
| _____ | | | |

### Food for Thought

_____
_____
_____

---

**Date:** _____

| Training | Time/Distance | Sets | Reps |
|----------|---------------|------|------|
| _____ | | | |
| _____ | | | |
| _____ | | | |
| _____ | | | |
| _____ | | | |

### Food for Thought

_____
_____
_____

**Date:**

| Training | Time/Distance | Sets | Reps |
|---|---|---|---|

**Food for Thought**

···························································································

**Date:**

| Training | Time/Distance | Sets | Reps |
|---|---|---|---|

**Food for Thought**

···························································································

**Date:**

| Training | Time/Distance | Sets | Reps |
|---|---|---|---|

**Food for Thought**

**Date:**

| Training | Time/Distance | Sets | Reps |
|---|---|---|---|
| | | | |
| | | | |
| | | | |
| | | | |
| | | | |

**Food for Thought**

................................................................

**Date:**

| Training | Time/Distance | Sets | Reps |
|---|---|---|---|
| | | | |
| | | | |
| | | | |
| | | | |
| | | | |

**Food for Thought**

................................................................

**Date:**

| Training | Time/Distance | Sets | Reps |
|---|---|---|---|
| | | | |
| | | | |
| | | | |
| | | | |
| | | | |

**Food for Thought**

**Date:**

| Training | Time/Distance | Sets | Reps |
|---|---|---|---|
| | | | |
| | | | |
| | | | |
| | | | |
| | | | |

### Food for Thought

_____

_____

_____

..................................................................................................

**Date:**

| Training | Time/Distance | Sets | Reps |
|---|---|---|---|
| | | | |
| | | | |
| | | | |
| | | | |
| | | | |

### Food for Thought

_____

_____

_____

### Workout Wrap-Up

| Accomplishments! | Notes |
|---|---|
| | |
| | |
| | |
| | |
| | |
| | |
| | |

*"I like long walks, especially when they are taken by people who annoy me."*

— Fred Allen, comedian

### Training Goals

Goals!

_____
_____
_____
_____
_____

**Date:** _____

| Training | Time/Distance | Sets | Reps |
|----------|---------------|------|------|
| _____ | | | |
| _____ | | | |
| _____ | | | |
| _____ | | | |
| _____ | | | |

### Food for Thought

_____
_____
_____

**Date:** _____

| Training | Time/Distance | Sets | Reps |
|----------|---------------|------|------|
| _____ | | | |
| _____ | | | |
| _____ | | | |
| _____ | | | |
| _____ | | | |

### Food for Thought

_____
_____
_____

**Date:**

| Training | Time/Distance | Sets | Reps |
|---|---|---|---|
| | | | |
| | | | |
| | | | |
| | | | |
| | | | |

**Food for Thought**

---

**Date:**

| Training | Time/Distance | Sets | Reps |
|---|---|---|---|
| | | | |
| | | | |
| | | | |
| | | | |
| | | | |

**Food for Thought**

---

**Date:**

| Training | Time/Distance | Sets | Reps |
|---|---|---|---|
| | | | |
| | | | |
| | | | |
| | | | |
| | | | |

**Food for Thought**

**Date:**

Training                                        Time/Distance          Sets  Reps

_____

_____

_____

_____

_____

**Food for Thought**

_____

_____

_____

..........................................................................................

**Date:**

Training                                        Time/Distance          Sets  Reps

_____

_____

_____

_____

_____

**Food for Thought**

_____

_____

_____

..........................................................................................

**Date:**

Training                                        Time/Distance          Sets  Reps

_____

_____

_____

_____

_____

**Food for Thought**

_____

_____

_____

**Date:**

| Training | Time/Distance | Sets | Reps |
|----------|---------------|------|------|

**Food for Thought**

·····················································································································

**Date:**

| Training | Time/Distance | Sets | Reps |
|----------|---------------|------|------|

**Food for Thought**

**Workout Wrap-Up**

Accomplishments!                    Notes

*"I don't believe for a second weightlifting is a sport. They pick up a heavy thing and put it down again. To me, that's indecision."*

— Paula Poundstone, comedian

## Training Goals
Goals!

---

| Date: | | | |
|---|---|---|---|

| Training | Time/Distance | Sets | Reps |
|---|---|---|---|
| | | | |
| | | | |
| | | | |
| | | | |
| | | | |

### Food for Thought

---

| Date: | | | |
|---|---|---|---|

| Training | Time/Distance | Sets | Reps |
|---|---|---|---|
| | | | |
| | | | |
| | | | |
| | | | |
| | | | |

### Food for Thought

**Date:**

| Training | Time/Distance | Sets | Reps |
|----------|---------------|------|------|
| | | | |
| | | | |
| | | | |
| | | | |
| | | | |

**Food for Thought**

................................................................................

**Date:**

| Training | Time/Distance | Sets | Reps |
|----------|---------------|------|------|
| | | | |
| | | | |
| | | | |
| | | | |
| | | | |

**Food for Thought**

................................................................................

**Date:**

| Training | Time/Distance | Sets | Reps |
|----------|---------------|------|------|
| | | | |
| | | | |
| | | | |
| | | | |
| | | | |

**Food for Thought**

**Date:**

Training                                    Time/Distance          Sets   Reps

_____

_____

_____

_____

_____

*Food for Thought*

_____

_____

_____

---

**Date:**

Training                                    Time/Distance          Sets   Reps

_____

_____

_____

_____

_____

*Food for Thought*

_____

_____

_____

---

**Date:**

Training                                    Time/Distance          Sets   Reps

_____

_____

_____

_____

_____

*Food for Thought*

_____

_____

_____

**Date:**

| Training | Time/Distance | Sets | Reps |
|----------|---------------|------|------|
| | | | |
| | | | |
| | | | |
| | | | |
| | | | |

**Food for Thought**

............................................................................................................

**Date:**

| Training | Time/Distance | Sets | Reps |
|----------|---------------|------|------|
| | | | |
| | | | |
| | | | |
| | | | |
| | | | |

**Food for Thought**

**Workout Wrap-Up**

| Accomplishments! | Notes |
|------------------|-------|
| | |
| | |
| | |
| | |
| | |
| | |
| | |

# Part III
# The Part of Tens

The 5th Wave   By Rich Tennant

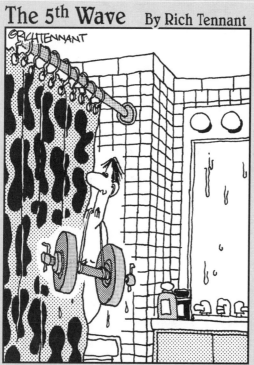

"Okay, I know I need to start working out. Now, can I please have my soap-on-a-rope back?"

## In this part . . .

*E*veryone loves a list, right? Well, the Part of Tens pages are like dessert, a few quick tips to help make exercising something that's not only good for you, but fun, too. Think of it as spinach salad with a crème brûlée chaser.

# Chapter 5

# Ten Weight Room Etiquette Tips

● ● ● ● ● ● ● ● ● ● ● ● ● ● ● ● ● ● ● ● ● ● ● ● ● ● ● ● ● ● ● ● ● ● ● ● ● ●

## In This Chapter

▶ Making friends with your fellow gym-goers

▶ Being polite

▶ Using a towel two different ways

● ● ● ● ● ● ● ● ● ● ● ● ● ● ● ● ● ● ● ● ● ● ● ● ● ● ● ● ● ● ● ● ● ● ● ● ● ●

*N*o, it's not dinner with Martha Stewart, but there is a definite code of conduct at the gym. Follow these rules and you'll fit right in.

## Rack Your Dumbbells

Remember how your mother used to pester you to put away your toys? The same applies at the gym. Once you're done with a dumbbell, return it to the rack in the place where it belongs so that your fellow gym-goers can find it.

## Unload Your Bar

You've finished your last rep on the bench press and you're done, right? Wrong. You still need to remove the plates from the bar and return them to the rack. And on a similar note, if you've added a half-plate weight to the stack on a machine, make sure to remove it when you're done.

# One Set and Out

This is the grown-up version of waiting your turn and playing nicely with others. If you're doing three sets on the chest press machine and there's someone hanging around waiting for it, you should voluntarily offer to let them "work in." That means alternating sets until you're both done. Simple? Great. Now do it.

# Observe Time Limits

The staff at the club doesn't put up those little signs just to test their graphic-arts skills. Just because there isn't someone peering over your shoulder doesn't mean there's no one waiting for the machine you're on. If the sign says there's a 20-minute time limit on the treadmill or stationary bike, believe it.

# Say "Please" and "Thank You"

When you're asking someone to spot for you, or if you can work in, a little attitude (or a little less attitude) goes a long way. Remember that those magic words still work, even in the gym.

# Wipe Down Your Equipment

Do you want to sit down on a soggy, sweaty hamstring curl machine? Then what makes you think that anyone else wants to do likewise? So carry a towel with you and wipe the machine down after you use it, or better yet, if the club provides them, use a paper towel and sanitizer to do it.

# Don't Leave Your Stuff Around

Most health clubs are crowded enough — all those machines take up plenty of space — without your plopping your coat and your gym bag right in the middle of the traffic pattern. If your bag is in the locker room, no one can trip over it.

# Use Your Locker

When you're heading for the shower, it's easy to dump your wet clothes on the floor where you shed them. It's also rude. That's why the club issued you a locker. Use it.

# Limit Your Shower Time

If you want to take a long, leisurely shower that hydrates every pore until you look like a prune, go right ahead . . . when you get home. At the club, limit your water time, because someone else is probably waiting.

# Be Modest

Yes, everyone knows you have a beautiful body. But that doesn't mean that you've got to show it to everyone in the locker room. Even a small towel goes a long way toward ridding the locker room of that nudist-colony vibe.

# Chapter 6

# Ten Top Weight-Lifting Songs

*O*ne of the coolest things about the gym is that you can listen to music while you work out. Here are ten songs that will provide a perfect soundtrack for your next trip to the gym.

## "The Weight," The Band

For some reason, this sepia-hued ballad makes me think of Thanksgiving. And how many extra sets I'll have to put in to work off that pumpkin pie. By the way, the Nazareth in the song isn't the city where Jesus lived, but the one in Pennsylvania where C.F. Martin Company makes guitars.

## "Carry That Weight," The Beatles

The last song on the last album the Beatles recorded, this song should remind you to slow down your sets. Take Paul's advice and "carry that weight a long time."

## "Something So Strong," Crowded House

The bouncy melody of this pure pop masterpiece will make three sets seem like one. And before long, the song's title will apply to you.

## "Press," Paul McCartney

A quick look at the rhyme scheme — stress rhymes with confess and mess — reveals that it's another one of Paul's silly love songs, but few can spin a tune like the cute Beatle.

## "Strong Enough," Sheryl Crow

In this put-up-or-shut-up ballad, Crow is talking about a different kind of strength, but that extra set builds character as well as muscle, right?

## "Pump It Up," Elvis Costello

Not to be confused with "Pump You Up," the driving beat of this New Wave classic makes it perfect for those high-rep sets.

## "We Can Work It Out," The Beatles

Get rid of the "It" and this title's all about hitting the gym. Put it back in and it's about explaining that three-hour trip to the gym to your significant other.

# "Strong Persuader," Robert Cray

Robert Cray's blues ballad is a cautionary tale about the power of physical attractiveness. So do another set, and use your newfound power wisely.

# "(Your Love Is Lifting Me) Higher and Higher," Jackie Wilson

This R&B milestone is inspiration concentrated in a two-and-a-half-minute package. Be sure to listen to the Jackie Wilson original; Rita Coolidge's cover will only make you want to lie down and take a nap.

# "Strength to Endure," The Ramones

This double-time rocker from New York's first family of punk is the musical equivalent of a double-espresso.

# Index

# Notes

# Notes

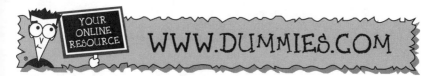

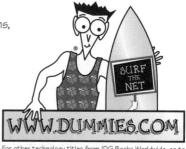

# IDG BOOKS WORLDWIDE BOOK REGISTRATION

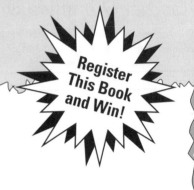
Register This Book and Win!

## We want to hear from you!

Visit **http://my2cents.dummies.com** to register this book and tell us how you liked it!

- ✔ Get entered in our monthly prize giveaway.

- ✔ Give us feedback about this book — tell us what you like best, what you like least, or maybe what you'd like to ask the author and us to change!

- ✔ Let us know any other *For Dummies*® topics that interest you.

Your feedback helps us determine what books to publish, tells us what coverage to add as we revise our books, and lets us know whether we're meeting your needs as a *For Dummies* reader. You're our most valuable resource, and what you have to say is important to us!

Not on the Web yet? It's easy to get started with *Dummies 101*®: *The Internet For Windows*® *98* or *The Internet For Dummies*®[3] at local retailers everywhere.

Or let us know what you think by sending us a letter at the following address:

*For Dummies* Book Registration
Dummies Press
10475 Crosspoint Blvd.
Indianapolis, IN 46256

...FOR DUMMIES™

BESTSELLING
BOOK SERIES

## Take the mystery out of exercising right!

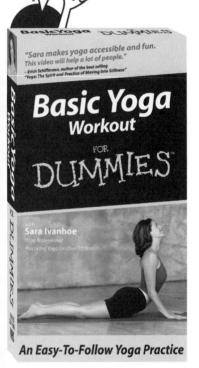

"Sara makes yoga accessible and fun. This video will help a lot of people."
– Erich Schiffmann, author of the best selling "Yoga: The Spirit and Practice of Moving into Stillness"

**Basic Yoga** Workout
FOR DUMMIES™

with Sara Ivanhoe
Yoga Professional
Practicing Yoga for Over 10 Years

*An Easy-To-Follow Yoga Practice*

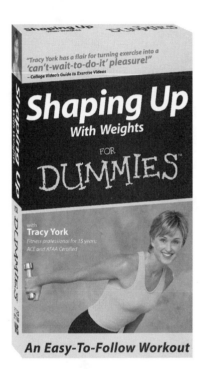

"Tracy York has a flair for turning exercise into a 'can't-wait-to-do-it' pleasure!"
– Collage Video's Guide to Exercise Videos

**Shaping Up** With Weights
FOR DUMMIES™

with Tracy York
Fitness professional for 15 years.
ACE and AFAA Certified

*An Easy-To-Follow Workout*

### *Introducing fitness videos for the rest of us!*
These un-intimidating exercise videos explain fitness techniques in easy-to-understand language. Not only can you re-shape your body with these videos — you may even change your mind about exercise.

**Available at retailers everywhere, or by calling (800) 546-1949.**

The ...For Dummies logo is a trademark, and Dummies Man, For Dummies, and ...For Dummies are registered trademarks of IDG Books Worldwide, Inc. Used by permission. All Rights Reserved.
©2000 by IDG Books Worldwide, Inc. All Rights Reserved.

Distributed By
Anchor Bay Entertainment, Inc.
1699 Stutz Dr., Troy, MI 48084
©2001 Anchor Bay Entertainment, Inc.
www.anchorbayentertainment.com

ANCHOR BAY
ENTERTAINMENT™